Throughout this book, the [author offers his own ideas]
and observations – as does Mark Occhipinti in this new,
updated edition. Both men's statements and opinions are
meant to serve only as an informational guide.

Persons who are in ill health should seek medical advice from a
doctor before embarking on any dietary program. Anyone
taking a prescribed medicine should not change nor terminate
that medication without consulting a physician. The facts and
the diet described in these pages are subject to different inter-
pretations and results. In other words, after reading this book,
you should use discretion and common sense.

TODD,

Always a pleasure -
meeting a member -

Best In Health,

Semper FI.

Mark Occhipinti

Dale Alexander's New Arthritis & Commonsense

VERMILION
LONDON

1 3 5 7 9 10 8 6 4 2

First published by Witkower Press Inc, USA

This revised edition published in the United Kingdom in 1999 by
Vermilion
an imprint of Ebury Press
Random House UK Ltd.
Random House
20 Vauxhall Bridge Road
London SW1V 2SA

Random House Australia (Pty) Limited.
20 Alfred Street, Milsons Point, Sydney,
New South Wales 2061, Australia

Random House New Zealand Limited
18 Poland Rd, Glenfield,
Auckland 10, New Zealand

Random House, South Africa (Pty) Limited
Box 2263, Rosebank 2121, South Africa

Random House UK Limited Reg. No. 954009

A CIP catalogue record for this book is available from the British
Library.

ISBN 0 09 181990 3

Printed and bound in Great Britain by
Mackays of Chatham PLC, Chatham, Kent

Papers used by Vermilion are natural, recyclable products made
from wood grown in sustainable forests.

Table of Contents

This book is dedicated to
. . . all suffers of arthritis, millions of you!

The doctor of the future will give no medicine, but will interest his patient in the case of the human frame, diet, and in the cause and prevention of disease.

Thomas A. Edison

Foreword

Dale 'The Codfather' Alexander is a powerful example of what one man can achieve through perseverance, enthusiasm and belief.

A self-educated man whose preaching was often at odds with the teaching of medical science, during his lifetime he nonetheless succeeded in making himself heard. And he could make a very loud noise indeed!

Alexander was undoubtedly ahead of his time. When his first book, *Arthritis and Common Sense*, was published in 1951, nutritional science was still in its infancy and medical science had nothing in its armory to combat the pain and joint stiffness – sometimes crippling – of arthritis. That something so simple, so familiar and so inexpensive as cod liver oil could make a difference was hard to swallow! Even now, when cod liver oil can call on an army of many thousands who swear it has transformed their lives, medicine still insists on prescribing strong drugs while relegating cod liver oil to the sidelines of arthritis treatment.

Although I was given cod liver oil as a child and came across it later at various points in my life, like Alexander, it took personal experience and the experience of colleagues and friends to convince me of the miracle that is cod liver oil. Through reading Dale Alexander's books I realised how many people could benefit from learning how to help themselves.

By the time Dale Alexander died in 1990, *Arthritis and Common Sense* had been translated into six languages and sold more than a million copies. Although four more books were published to keep pace with the advance of scientific knowledge, research into natural therapies since his death has come up with a wealth of evidence to prove that cod liver oil does work and to explain how and why it is so effective. I have included, where relevant, these new findings and some comments of my own. More than anything, they demonstrate how much he knew before science was prepared to endorse it.

Dale Alexander had a vision. With this book I hope to reach more people with his simple self-help messages, and, at last, gain recognition for his single-minded crusade on behalf of the millions of arthritis sufferers in the world.

My Story

My first cod liver oil memory involves my Norwegian grandmother. Every day she would give me a spoonful of a dark liquid that smelled bad and tasted even worse. She told me that it was good for me.

Although I was always a healthy child, I was short, plump and plain and came in for constant teasing and bullying at school. This was my motivation to become as strong, muscular, powerful and fit as I could be. I was determined never to be bullied again!

I set out to become a competitive power-lifter and body-builder and researched how best I could become stronger and gain more muscle mass.

As part of my research I bought books on nutrition and the role of various specialist nutritional products. The more I read, the more I wanted to learn.

While working my way through college, I helped out in a health food store at weekends. The store stocked many books on nutrition and health, one of which was on cod liver oil by Dale Alexander. Following my childhood experience, I was fascinated by his theories, but at that time in my life I simply stored the information at the back of my mind.

Later, however, when I turned to outdoor work as a

commercial clammer/fisherman to earn extra money, cod liver oil again entered my life – although not quite as Dale Alexander recommended! During the winter months along the New Jersey coastline the cold and wind really pound the body. I started to use cod liver oil on my skin (especially my face) when I was on the water to protect my skin from chapping.

Following graduation, I began working for a company selling fish oil capsules (primarily cod liver oil) to physicians. Because I needed background knowledge to be convincing in my job, I read up on cod liver and fish oils and the role of omega-3 fatty acids. Once again I was impressed by Dale Alexander's pioneering research into cod liver oil but, being young, fit and healthy, still thought it wasn't for someone like me.

It was almost ten years later that I had good personal reasons to be grateful for reading Dale Alexander's books. As a result of multiple weight-lifting injuries, I was suffering from severe shoulder pain. I decided to try a course of cod liver oil and, over a six-week period, noted that both shoulders progressively responded to the treatment. I took no other medication. Thanks to cod liver oil, I was able to resume my training and progress to even heavier weights with no pain. On my recommendation, several of my colleagues tried the treatment and reported similarly good results.

This was when I became hooked on investigating the science behind cod liver oil. I learned that researchers from all over the world were at last uncovering the evidence to prove what Dale Alexander had discovered by his own experience and by talking to a handful of enlightened practitioners.

The evidence for heart health was so strong that it convinced me to take low-level fish oils (one 200mg capsule daily) to protect against heart disease. Evidently the dosage was too low to correct an ever-increasing problem that I was experiencing. Red blotches appeared on both my chest and the base of my neck and on my arms. At times they would itch and cause embarrassment if I had to remove my shirt at the beach or in the locker room at the gym. My doctor put me on cortisone creams, which were both expensive and had unwelcome side-effects. Within a week of my coming off the cream, the blotches would return, sometimes with a vengeance.

However, I found an unexpected and surprising answer to my problem. When the shoulder complaint returned after overenthusiastic training, I followed Dale Alexander's recipe for one tablespoon of cod liver oil liquid daily mixed with orange juice. After only eight weeks I noticed that not only had the shoulder pain 95 per cent gone but my skin condition had cleared up. I had discontinued the cortisone creams in disgust more than six months previously. Not long after that I found several studies that discussed using omega-3 fatty acids in fish oils for the treatment of eczema and other skin complaints.

I told a close friend who suffered terribly from eczema with large blotches all over her arms, hands and torso. Within several weeks on the Dale Alexander program her skin had cleared up remarkably.

Out of my own experiences I have developed a deep respect for a man who, with no formal training, was able to cut his way through the cant and ritual of the medical profession – and win. Although there is still a long way to go, more and more doctors and scientists are turning to dietary solutions in the search for optimum health and in the fight against disease and debilitating conditions associated with ageing. I believe Dale Alexander played a major part in this.

I am grateful for his teaching and proud to be associated with his work. I sincerely hope and believe you will be helped to better health if you follow Dale Alexander's advice. However, do heed the warnings on page 1. A book can only advise in general terms, whereas your doctor knows you and your medical history.

Mark Occhipinti

Chapter I
Dale Alexander – In His Own Words

You and I have a common interest. Our goal is to resist and repel the painful misery of arthritis.

As I write this new book, my purpose is to bring you more facts and more answers – to help you conquer this illness.

Here are the key facts, important evidence I have gathered during the past 30 years.

My experiences – my worldwide travels since 1951 – have convinced me that millions of arthritics can benefit from the ideas I shall now set forth in this book.

When a man spends an entire lifetime studying just one disease, certainly he must learn some valuable information about that ailment. It is my hope that you will seriously consider the testimony which I now offer. I shall attempt to prove that arthritis is a constitutional disorder, not just an illness which causes aching, swollen joints.

Many of the chapters in this book will also bear witness to the fact that arthritis can be affected by good nutrition and proper diet. I will quote many physicians and scientists who believe as I do regarding certain dietary factors. You can now read about all the latest research*, and evaluate it. Then, you can act – on the basis of your own judgement and common sense.

*This book was first published in 1951 and revised in 1987. In 1999, I have commented where new research findings either confirm, change or cast doubt on Dale Alexander's views.

I openly admit that my dietary program, designed to alleviate arthritis, is a theory. But I shall submit so many relevant facts, from so many sources, that you may agree with my logic and my conclusions.

Before you begin to read this book, let's talk about credibility. You have the right to ask: 'Who is this man, Dale Alexander? Where did he come from? What are his credentials, and is he qualified to discuss arthritis with any degree of authority?'

My reputation, as an author and lecturer, dates back to 1951 when the first volume of *Arthritis and Common Sense* was published. I never expected that the public response would be so overwhelming. I am deeply grateful that so many people saw merit in that book, and told their friends.

Now, more than 1,200,000 copies are in print, distributed throughout the world. I am humble, in awe of that total. Because I never intended to become an 'author'. I just wanted to write a diary of facts about a remarkable experience which happened to my mother. She was a victim of crippling arthritis. By changing her diet, my mother recovered her health. Perhaps other people could benefit by reading her story. That was the simple intent of my first book.

Readers soon found that my dietary program was equally effective for them. The good news spread – and, quite by accident, suddenly I was catapulted into the role of being a 'famous' author.

At first, the only way people heard about my book was by word of mouth. A relative or a friend was feeling better, thanks to some new method of eating.

Victims of arthritis, scattered in cities and towns across America, began reporting that their pain had receded. They were enjoying better health.

People, by the thousands, began talking about Dale Alexander. Was it possible that, somehow, he had found a partial solution to arthritic ailments?

The medical profession was quick to discount 'the Alexander approach'. They announced it was too simple an answer. 'Diet to combat arthritis? Nonsense!' Many doctors told their patients that the book was not responsible for improving health. 'You are merely experiencing a period of spontaneous remission – the pain relief is only temporary.'

But so many people reported long-lasting relief, there was no way to 'bury' this encouraging news story. National magazines began writing articles and soon I found myself being interviewed on the major television networks.

When I appeared on *The Arthur Godfrey Show* it drew an avalanche of mail. Millions of arthritics had questions to ask – and all the major TV programs invited me to respond. I went 'on the air' with Mike Douglas, Merv Griffin, Johnny Carson.

So many people wrote letters – after my interview on *The Tonight Show* that the producers asked me to return for a second time. That night, David Brenner was the guest host. We mixed in some humor, along with the serious suggestions about diet and nutrition.

I've always been just a quiet man, from a small town in Connecticut. So those TV 'talk shows' were exciting events for me. I was the 'unknown author' who was swept into the spotlight, unawares.

The so-called 'fame' which I have now acquired is not important. But it does serve one purpose. Now I receive many more requests to lecture about arthritis . . . and that is my primary goal in life.

If I can teach about nutrition-speak before new audiences, throughout the world – I shall travel this earth to help arthritics.

My Quest For Knowledge... How It All Began

To learn everything possible about rheumatic illness, my early research was done in libraries. I studied medical literature, dozens of books. Many of them contained facts on arthritis, but the volumes were so ancient they had been forgotten and 'lost' in the archives. With the help of librarians – in Hartford, Boston and New York – I traced the history of this illness through the centuries.

I read about many remedies which had been tried in the past. But none of these 'cures' had been truly successful, none of them had caused permanent relief from pain.

Time after time, as I was reading all these reports and scientific papers, the same two words reappeared constantly: 'etiology [cause] unknown.' No matter what type of arthritis was being discussed, the doctors would write that the real cause of this disease was still unknown.

After long months of searching in these medical libraries, however, I did find some clues. I saw a pattern of facts starting to develop.

It became obvious to me that arthritics were suffering from a lack of oil-bearing foods. Their bodies were 'drying out' too often and too soon.

Dryness in the linings of their joints was the main problem to be solved. If I could find a way to lubricate tissues surrounding the joints, perhaps I could end my mother's pain-racked ordeal.

Back in those days, before World War II, her ailment was simply called 'rheumatism' – and she had a hopeless case. 'Etiology unknown.'

My first attempts to help her involved cod liver oil, and little else. But she did respond, remarkably well. Since then, I have expanded and improved my dietary program, based on added research and the wealth of information I have gathered from actual arthritics.

Later in this book, I shall offer an entire chapter which gives a detailed description of how lubrication occurs within your body. I will discuss digestion, absorption and assimilation. These are the three keystones. What I say happens to the foods you digest does occur. My theory is physiologically possible . . . and I'll give you a pictorial map of where the oils travel.

Phase Two... My Education Among Actual Arthritics

Most physicians must practice medicine in just one city or town. They open an office, and they can see only a few hundred patients per year. I enjoy a special advantage, because I have met thousands of arthritics, face to face, and I have listened to their specific questions about rheumatic ailments.

Everywhere I travel, the people who attend my lectures tell me about their personal experiences – how they have fought their own battles, what methods they have used as they try to 'cure' their arthritis.

I have learned from all these encounters and discussions. It is possible that I have talked with more arthritics than any other man alive. All these lectures – spanning 30 years – have also allowed me to ask questions. When people told me about some new treatment they had tried, I would promptly investigate its powers to heal.

While preparing to write this book, I leafed through some of my scrapbooks. They are filled with newspaper clippings, a record of my travels. What marvelous memories! My early lecture tours took me to more than 95 cities throughout the United States.

I remember speaking in bookstores, on college campuses, in church basements, and in huge auditoriums. When it was announced that I would lecture in St. Petersburg, Florida, no hall was large enough. The event had to be held in a public park. That day, the total attendance was more than 6,000 people.

Another milestone was my first trip to Canada. The lecture took place, on campus, at the University of British Columbia.

Jet aircraft makes any journey possible. I flew to South Africa, traveled to Johannesburg. There, I spoke before 90 doctors, residents and interns at the University of Witwatersand.

Next came invitations to lecture in Australia. I accepted immediately, and took off for Melbourne.

The friendly people throughout Australia gave me a warm welcome. They were eager to hear my views about arthritis – because this disease has swept across that continent, worsening every year. I was questioned closely at the University of Sydney. That nation also broadcasts an Australian edition of *Meet The Press* – and I appeared on that program. The telecast became an excellent debate, as I argued on behalf of better nutrition.

Other clippings pasted in my scrapbook describe my lectures in England, Ireland and Wales. I have flown to London three separate times – in order to meet with readers of my book. I toured the British Isles, including Scotland, lecturing in a dozen different cities.

Arthritis has now invaded every nation around the world. This harrowing illness has spread across oceans – to every outpost of civilization. It has even struck people who live on islands in the South Seas.

I went to New Zealand, because arthritics there needed help. In that country, I lectured in Dunedin, at the Otago Medical School.

Incidentally, a purported 'cure' for arthritis has surfaced in New Zealand. I have checked it out, and I'll report my findings in this book (see page 28). The treatment is being developed by a marine pharmacologist. Experiments indicate that shellfish may contain therapeutic substances. Being tested are mussels grown in the waters near Auckland, New Zealand.

As I mention these travels of mine, I am not just reminiscing. There's a point to be made. I want you to know the extent of my past education.

I circle the globe, on a constant quest for the truth about arthritis. I talk with surgeons, and pathologists, and biochemists. I visit laboratories and clinics, attend conferences and seminars.

Yes, I am self-educated. And I'm proud of it!

The most significant fact is that I have met with thousands of people who had arthritis. They experienced this painful affliction personally. Bless them all! They gave me their knowledge, to share with you.

So I shall write this book, hoping to shed some light on a difficult topic. There's a certain clipping, in my scrapbook, which describes my one goal in life. The editors of *Healthview Newsletter* interviewed me, and here's what they wrote:

Dale Alexander is a layman who became interested in arthritis back in the late 1920s, when his mother was stricken with the disease.

'I saw her suffer,' he says, 'for 10 long years. I know the damage arthritis can do to a person and to her family.

'Over the years, her condition gradually deteriorated. The swelling increased. Her knees began to give out. Her fingers became so stiff she could barely open or close her hands. The pain was so constant and intense you could hardly say she was living any more – she was barely existing.

'I felt heartbroken to see her suffering – and frustrated because there was nothing I could do about it. It was so maddening that one day something snapped inside of me. I had to do something, anything, to help her. I couldn't watch her suffering any more. From that moment on, I've devoted my life to helping my mother – and all arthritic sufferers like her.'

Chapter II
A Typical Interview: Probing My Views

Journalists – the working press – are not admired when they ask hard-hitting questions. Any author who agrees to an interview should certainly expect to be interrogated closely.

I welcome such sessions, where the newspapermen or magazine writers demand honest answers. They want confirmation, added facts, to support every statement you make. That's fine, the way it should be.

For the most part, the interviewers I have faced have been fair-minded and friendly. But once in a while I encounter a writer who is anti-nutrition and says so from the start.

Let me give you an example of how it feels to be interviewed 'in depth', when the questions are tough, and nobody pulls any punches.

One reason I respect *Healthview Newsletter* is the caliber of their editors. They search hard for news, so they compiled a list of far-reaching questions. 'Find out what makes Alexander tick. Put him through the mill.'

For this special interview, I traveled to them. Ready to meet, I arrived at their editorial offices in Charlottesville, Virginia. They were skeptical, I guess. They began by asking a 'loaded' question:

Healthview Newsletter: Obviously, you had a good measure of success with your mother, or you wouldn't have published your book. How did you, as a layman, with no medical background at all, come to develop a successful program where thousands of doctors have failed?

Alexander: I started off by reading everything about arthritis I could get my hands on. I began to haunt the medical libraries. At first, I couldn't find anything of value. Everything I came across my mother had already tried – heat, ointments (you can't imagine how many different kinds), drugs, exercises. They had even extracted her teeth – a popular treatment at the time. But none of these had given her more than mild, temporary relief – so I knew I had to go further.

Healthview Newsletter: What did you do?

Alexander: I kept going. My research went in two directions – interestingly enough, they were opposite.

On the one hand, I pursued all the latest medical findings and current research. On the other hand, I started digging into the past, into forgotten 'remedies' and 'folk cures'.

Needless to say, the great bulk of the material was worthless. But, in an old medical book, published in 1855, I came upon one old-time folk remedy that was to prove to be the lost 'key' to solving the problems of arthritis.

The book was by a medical doctor, a Dr. L. J. deJong, who had tested it in his daily practice. He had found that it worked better than anything else he had ever heard of.

The doctor had no idea of why it worked, but the more I thought about it, the more sense it made to me. It seemed to fit the facts about arthritis – which we'll get into later. But back then, what was very important to me was that the remedy was completely safe*.

---

*Cod liver oil contains four important nutrients: Vitamin A, Vitamin D, the omega-3 essential fatty acids EPA (eicosapentaenoic acid) and DHA (docosahexaenoic acid). Because the two vitamins are fat soluble and can be stored in the body, in very high quantities they can be toxic. For this reason, people are warned not to take cod liver oil in high doses. However, fears about Vitamin A and D toxicity and overdose from cod liver oil are greatly exaggerated. To approach toxic levels through cod liver oil intake, you would have to take the equivalent of 150ml (half a standard-size bottle) daily for six months.

It could do only good: at worst my mother's condition would be unchanged. So I spoke with her about it. She decided to give it a fair try.

Healthview Newsletter: What happened?

Alexander: At first, nothing.

Then, after 10 weeks, the first in a series of curious changes came over her. Her hair, which had been lifeless and dry, began to recover its luster and sheen.

During the twelfth week, another change occurred. Her skin, always very dry, became soft and supple.

Skin condition is one of the recognized indicators of essential fatty acid deficiency. As cod liver oil supplies the omega-3 DHA and EPA fatty acids, it is not surprising that Alexander's mother's skin improved.

The omega-3s also help in cases of dandruff. Vitamin A is known as the skin vitamin and it is also recommended for strong and healthy hair. She would also have noticed an improvement in her nails.

Dale Alexander reports that his mother began to notice these visible effects of taking cod liver oil after 10 weeks and joint improvement after five months. <u>Cod liver oil usually needs to be taken for six months for the benefits to be felt.</u> Patience is important.

Next she discovered a new sensation in her ears. She found that, for the first time in years, she was developing ear wax, which is normal in a healthy person.

The last, and most notable, change was the one we had been seeking all along: relief from her arthritic condition. In the middle of the fifth month – that's quite some time – it happened. Her fingers and arms began to lose their swelling and stiffness. The pain began to recede. Next, her knees began to feel better, and finally her back.

Once the first sign of improvement had begun, the whole process moved quite rapidly. Before long there was pain-free motion! After so many years of suffering, her long ordeal was over.

We were so happy, we cried.

Healthview Newsletter: What was that remedy you gave her?

Alexander: Oddly enough, it was plain old cod liver oil. It sounds like an unlikely solution, doesn't it? But you ought to see what it can do for arthritis.

What cod liver oil does is to increase the quality of the joint fluid. You see, the basic cause of arthritis is that the lubricating fluid in the joints gets too thin. It doesn't lubricate properly. So, naturally, your joints become stiff and difficult to move.

When human joints lack the proper lubricating fluid, the various parts of the joint – the cartilage, the joint lining, the bony parts – begin to rub and grind against one another. There's friction, then stiffness, then irritation, and then finally inflammation. That's just what the word arthritis means: inflammation of the joints. 'Arth' means joint and 'itis' means inflammation.

Incidentally, it doesn't matter what kind of arthritis you have, they all respond to cod liver oil. The reason for this is that all arthritis – regardless of the symptoms – has the same basic cause: poorly lubricated joints. It's just that each person reacts differently.

For example, if friction causes the cartilage to wear away, we call it osteoarthritis. If it's the joint lining that suffers, it's rheumatoid arthritis. No matter what the symptoms, cod liver oil will help.

Healthview Newsletter: That's an interesting theory. Do you have any evidence to back it up?

Alexander: I certainly do. I didn't just read a few articles on cod liver oil, and run out and publish a book. I knew I had a big responsibility – both to the public and to the medical profession.

I knew I was definitely on to something, but I realized I had to back up my theories with solid, indisputable evidence. Otherwise, why should anyone pay attention to me?

As soon as my mother was back on her feet, I returned to the medical libraries to pick up where I had left off.

I found a report in Dr. Ralph Pemberton's book, *The Medical Management of Arthritis*, which showed that normal people have joint fluid that's over 15 times as thick and viscous as the fluid in arthritic joints. What a difference! It shows the tremendous variation in joint fluid between a healthy person and an arthritic.

I learned that the joint linings can accept nutritional oils directly from the bloodstream. I also learned that cartilage – the tissue next to the bone – could absorb these oils from the lining, through osmosis.

Editor's note: In this interview, the questions by *Healthview Newsletter* have been quoted exactly word for word. The answers, given by Alexander, have been edited slightly, primarily to condense his replies and conserve space in this book.

Healthview Newsletter: Has cod liver oil ever been tested by the medical profession?

Alexander: Many times. Medical literature is full of accounts of its use as a folk remedy two hundred years back in the treatment of arthritis.

More recently, in 1920 to be precise, cod liver oil was tested and approved by Dr. Ralph Pemberton of the University of Pennsylvania. He was one of the leading rheumatologists of all time. The highest honor a rheumatologist can receive today is to be called upon to give the annual Pemberton Lecture on Rheumatology. That gives you an idea of the esteem in which Dr. Pemberton is held.

Dr. Pemberton tested cod liver oil on hundreds of arthritic patients. He reported his findings in his report entitled, 'Studies on Arthritis in the Army Based on Four Hundred Cases', which appeared in the *Archives of Internal Medicine* (March, 1920).

After thorough testing, Dr. Pemberton concluded that cod liver oil was effective in eliminating the pain, stiffness and swelling of chronic arthritis. This is quite an endorsement, coming from a man like Dr. Pemberton.

I know the theory works, because over the years, I've received thousands of letters from people throughout America – and later around the world – who have tried cod liver oil.

For instance, I received a letter from a woman in St. Petersburg, Florida. Let me read it to you.

She said:

Dear Dale Alexander,

Twenty-five years ago, I was unable to walk. Every joint in my body was aching. My husband had to carry me up the stairs. . . . My doctors told me I would eventually have to be in a wheelchair.

I read your book and took cod liver oil. In one month, I was able to walk and work. The pain was gone. Now and then I go off the cod liver oil and the pain comes back. So, I go back to it and I am alright again, thank God. If it were not for your book, I would today be a complete invalid.

Author's comment: I showed that letter, and others like it, to the editors who were interviewing me. They saw written proof that cod liver oil is a viable weapon against arthritis. People write to me all the time – sincere, thankful letters – and they inspire me to continue my research work.

I never resent it when journalists express some doubt about my dietary theories. They have a right to demand medical confirmation and supporting facts. The writers are being vigilant, protecting their readers.

You may have noticed that this interview – with *Healthview Newsletter* – contained repeated questions which were asked with a tone of skepticism. They were 'grilling' me. In fact, this was their very last query: 'What does the medical profession think of your program?'

I replied, quite frankly, that some doctors are still attacking my nutritional claims. But attitudes are changing, in my favor. This was my final answer:

I think it's only a matter of time before the medical profession will turn to diet as a real 'cure' for arthritis. It happened with insulin. Not too many years ago, doctors relied on insulin to control diabetes. Now, they recognize diet as an accepted and preferred method of treatment. I predict the same thing will happen with arthritis.

The future outlook is encouraging. For readers of this book, I shall list the most beneficial foods. But in the next chapter, I give you all the facts on cod liver oil.

Because arthritis is such a widespread and debilitating condition – affecting more and more people as a result of the ageing population and the increasing dependence on fast and processed foods – it has attracted a great deal of global attention from medical science and generated many hundreds of clinical trials and research. Since Dale Alexander discovered cod liver oil through personal experience, trial and error, research has provided a wealth of evidence to support much of his thinking. Using oil to produce improvements in inflammatory conditions such as arthritis would have seemed highly implausible to doctors twenty years ago, but is now widely accepted.

Cod liver oil contains high levels of the omega-3 essential fatty acids DHA (docosahexaenoic acid) and EPA (eicosapentaenoic acid). (Essential fatty acids were at one time known as Vitamin F, which may be simpler to pronounce but is too simplistic a term to be useful.) Although discovered decades ago, the importance of these long-chain polyunsaturated fatty acids was, incredibly, overlooked until as recently as the early 1970s.

It was discovered that the omega-3s, among their many other health benefits, are powerful anti-inflammatory agents. They cannot be manufactured by the body, they must come from diet. Omega-3 vegetable sources do exist (flaxseed, walnuts, and rapeseed, for example) but the body is invariably unable to convert the omega-3 linolenic acid they supply into the useful DHA and EPA forms. They are much less likely to produce real benefits.

Oily fish, fish oil supplements and cod liver oil are almost the only readily available sources of omega-3 DHA and EPA that reduce levels of potent chemicals (leukotrienes, certain prostaglandins and cytokines) involved in many inflammatory conditions, including arthritis.

Chapter III
Cod Liver Oil: The Best Solution

K nowing the correct foods to eat, and having a truly balanced diet, are important. But the speed of your recovery will definitely depend on cod liver oil. It can be your greatest ally. As an anti-arthritic agent, this oily solution has no equal!

Until now, like most people, you have probably ignored cod liver oil. You have tried to forget the fishy substance. It was something your mother poured into a spoon and forced you to swallow.

'As a medication, this oil doesn't belong in the Space Age. It's an old-fashioned remedy. Used by my grandmother, for her aches and pains.'

I hear remarks like these almost every day. By reputation, cod liver oil is just an ancient cure-all. People sometimes smile, bemused, when I recommend they try it. So I intend to write an entire chapter on this matter. Perhaps if you know the complete history of cod liver oil, you'll respect it more.

No matter where arthritis strikes in your body, the lubricating properties of this oil can alleviate the problem. It's a grim fact, but doctors can now diagnose more than 100 ailments as being some form of 'arthritic' disease.

Further investigations into the roots and courses of disease would now put this figure nearer 200.

Your first step, on the road to recovery, is to learn what type of arthritis is ruining your life. Know your enemy. With so many different varieties to choose from, only a qualified physician or a trained rheumatologist can determine the exact nature of your illness.

I have always recommended that any person who is ill should consult a doctor for a complete physical examination. Describe your arthritic symptoms to him, ask him all the questions you can concerning the form of treatment he proposes. (If you wish, show him this book. See what he thinks about cod liver oil.)

If your doctor wants to 'study up on the subject' before rendering his verdict you might suggest that he read a certain medical paper. The special report was written by a physician from the Department of Pediatrics, Yale University School of Medicine. The title is: 'The History of Cod Liver Oil as a Remedy'.

I might add, most respectfully, that the author was a woman, a lady doctor. Her research work was monumental. She traced the use of cod liver oil, and discovered it has been effective as a medicine for hundreds of years. I extend my congratulations to her – to Ruth Guy, M.D. – for a job well done.

Historic Highlights, Down Through The Centuries

America was fighting a war in 1776, and there's no record that George Washington took cod liver oil on any regular basis. But, in England, physicians were already prescribing the oil for chronic rheumatism. In 1771 it was entered in the British Pharmacopaeia.

Old documents state that patients were given cod liver oil at the Manchester Infirmary . . . so frequently that the institution used 'near a hogshead [about 52.5 imperial gallons] annually'.

Cod liver oil has been used as a medicine for centuries. The fishermen of Iceland, Greenland, Norway and Scotland have used it for thousands of years, but the first extensive clinical tests seem to have been made by Samuel Kay, a physician at the Manchester Infirmary from 1752 to 1784. He gave doses of cod liver oil to people suffering from bone diseases and rheumatism. Following reports of Kay's work, a German physician, Schenk, did further research and the publication of his experiences led to a wider appreciation of the medicinal value of cod liver oil. Gradually it began to be used, not haphazardly in the treatment of almost any kind of ailment, but specifically for diseases related to malnutrition. But nobody knew why it worked.

At the beginning of this century, doctors realized that the oil was a curative for rickets – a disease rife at that time. But not until the 1920s was Vitamin D identified as the active ingredient. It was this revelation that attracted the serious scientific attention and research that was in part responsible for the discovery of the omega-3 fatty acids. Research is still finding out more about these valuable health nutrients.

In 1807, a Dr. Bardsley of that same infirmary gave his findings on cod liver oil. He reported: 'It has operated in a manner so decidedly beneficial as to excite astonishment.'

In 1910, according to Dr. Guy, an expert named Rosenstern made a very valid statement. He wrote: 'Cod liver oil is in the forefront of children's remedies. For long it has been struggling against the skepticism of exact science.'

For anyone who might still be skeptical, I have a true story to tell. Let me recall an historic event which happened during World War II.

When Hitler had London under siege, the British Government feared that food supplies would be cut off, endangering the health of babies and toddlers. So they enacted a law to provide all children with a 'ration' of two key products. Throughout the war, these two crucial items were supplied to families.

What were the two chosen products, considered so vital? Orange juice and cod liver oil.

> Orange juice and cod liver oil were provided free to children under five, pregnant women and nursing mothers. Orange juice was known to be a valuable source of Vitamin C when fresh produce was often hard to come by (it was already well accepted that Vitamin C was a daily health essential). Cod liver oil was supplied essentially as a source of Vitamin D at a time when many children were afflicted by the bone-deforming disease, rickets, caused by Vitamin D deficiency. They were doing more nutritional good than they knew.

Today, scientific laboratories in the United States have the capability to analyze oil-bearing foods. I must report, however, that the most extensive research work on cod liver oil has been carried out by British workers in the clinics and hospitals of Europe.

They have established the importance of certain poly-unsaturated fatty acids – including EPA and DHA – which are known to be present in cod liver oil.

Would you like to read my detailed description of their highly technical experiments? I could explain that EPA is eicosapentaenoic acid and DHA is docosahexaenoic acid. But I believe that their favorable effect in our fight against arthritis ought to be stated in very simple terms. I shall try to do so, later in this book, when I discuss 'osmosis' and how your body can absorb beneficial oils.

For now, just let me emphasize that the world of science is actively studying cod liver oil. Since 1978 there has been more major research published on this subject than for the previous 50 years!

The Omega-3 Story

Once upon a time there was something in diet described as 'Vitamin F'. The term now used is essential fatty acids (EFAs). Like vitamins, EFAs are essential to life and health and must be obtained from diet.

Essential fatty acids are the building blocks of the membranes of all the cells in the body. Without them, our cells simply cannot grow or function properly. Cell walls become rigid and metabolism is impaired.

As well as having a role in the immune system, energy reserves and vitamin transportation, EFAs are the raw material from which the body makes prostaglandins – hormone-like chemicals which control such vital bodily processes as blood clotting and inflammation.

There are about 20 essential fatty acids and all but two – omega-6 and omega-3 – can be produced by the human body. Omega-6 and omega-3 EFAs are polyunsaturated fatty acids that can only be obtained from diet. They should be consumed in a balance whose ideal has been generally accepted as two or three times more omega-6 than omega-3.

As long as the body is provided with the proper balance of omega-3 and omega-6 fatty acids along with the right combination of vitamins and minerals, it will produce beneficial prostaglandins that promote good health. However, as a result of increased consumption of polyunsaturated vegetable oils and margarines over the past few decades, the balance is quite out of

OMEGA-3 METABOLIC PATHWAY

Alpha-linolenic acid
(ALA)
18:3 Ω3

Walnuts and walnut
oil, pumpkin
seeds, linseed
(flaxseed) oil

delta-6 desaturase
enzyme activity

delta-5 desaturase
enzyme activity

Eicosapentaenoic acid
(EPA)
20:5 Ω3

Prostaglandins
(PG) series 3

delta-4 desaturase
enzyme activity*

Oily fish (eg
mackerel, salmon,
herring), cod liver
and fish oils

Docosahexaenoic acid
(DHA)
22:6 Ω3

Prostacyclins
(biological regulators)

*alternative pathways have been proposed

kilter. Western diets of today contain something in the order of seven or eight times more omega-6 than omega-3. As a result, our cells choose to produce a prostaglandin that is pro-inflammatory, encourages blood clotting with potentially disastrous consequences, and can lead to depression and mental illness.

In the beginning

In the 1970s, researchers noted that the Inuit peoples native to Greenland enjoyed remarkable cardiovascular health despite a diet heavily reliant on seal and whalemeat (blubber) and fatty fish. Given what was already known about fat and heart disease, this apparent contradiction led British and Danish scientists to study what became known as 'the Eskimo diet'. This research resulted in the identification the omega-3 fatty acids which in turn spawned more studies into the health benefits and effects of these newly-discovered nutrients. Many of the subsequent studies reported positive findings and generated a spate of further trials and an interest which continues to this day.

To date, the omega-3 EFAs have been strongly associated with:

* Protection against heart disease and thrombotic (blood clot) stroke
* Relief of inflammatory conditions, principally arthritis, psoriasis, Crohn's disease
* Prevention of certain cancers including cancer of the colon and those linked to hormonal activity such as breast and prostate cancers
* Multiple sclerosis
* Depression and schizophrenia

It has also been established that the omega-3 EFAs are important to brain development in the unborn and new-born and to healthy brain function into old age.

Best sources
Marine: Salmon, herring, trout, mackerel, sardines, pilchard, eel, anchovies, tuna.
Vegetable: Pumpkin seed, canola, chia candlenut, leafy green vegetables (variable amounts)
There is no doubt that the best sources of the omega-3s are all of marine origin. Although some plants do supply omega-3 nutrients (walnuts and walnut oil, purslane, flaxseeds and oil (linseed), some pulses and soyabean oil), the enzyme needed for prostaglandin conversion seldom works efficiently. The majority of researchers believe that the only reliable sources of omega-3 are cod liver oil and other fish oils. And, of course, cod liver oil also contains the Vitamin D so highly prized by Dale Alexander and the many nutritionists who followed in his footsteps.

The Russians Are Coming!

They have gone into battle. The Soviet Union is our ally this time, in the war against arthritis.

Russian scientists have already conducted some valuable experiments, a series of medical tests which may lead to a cure for rheumatic illness.

Arthritis is an affliction which transcends all political boundaries. If the Soviets can be the first to discover an effective remedy, their success will be deserved. Because they have been quietly working on the problem for at least three decades.

I recently obtained a special report, translated from Russian, concerning research work which was done by I. I. Khvorostukhin from the Stanilslausk Medical Institute.

After studying this material I was amazed. The report revealed that the Russians were experimenting with cod liver oil as far back as 1961!

What the Russian scientists tried to establish was this: 'Can damaged joint cartilage repair itself and be regenerated?'

If victims of arthritis could be given the gift of healthy cartilage, these laboratory tests would be of historic importance.

Unfortunately, the Russians employed a technique which I deplore. They performed operations on 22 dogs. Each animal was inflicted with bone cartilage injuries in both knee joints.

I condemn most experiments using animals.

Next, the Russians injected cod liver oil – hoping to stimulate the regeneration of cartilage. I have never proposed injecting the oil in animals or humans.

For nearly six months, the dogs were observed and microscopic studies were made. Some regeneration of cartilage was reported. But, for better results, they should change the testing procedures. Next time, experiment with human beings – and let them take cod liver oil orally.

We Travel On: From Moscow To The South Pacific

For a vacation, to relax in the sun, let's visit the tropical islands near New Zealand. Last time I was there I had no time to enjoy life. The people of New Zealand kept me busy answering questions about arthritis. They are fighting to banish this illness.

As an example of their efforts, let me tell you a fish story, a shellfish story. This is the saga of New Zealand Green-Lipped Mussels.

A scientist named John E. Croft has derived an extract from mussels. The product is taken orally, and some arthritics have reported therapeutic results.

It is interesting to note that, once again, the remedy is related to marine life. I say codfish can yield the necessary oils. He proclaims that mussels hold the answer.

Experiments continue in New Zealand, with mussels being

grown in aquatic farms. I am not surprised by these developments. In the past, chemists have analyzed shark oil, whale oil, and dozens of alternatives. None can match the advantages of cod liver oil.

Millions of years ago, man evolved from marine life. Senior academics and scientists are now seriously proposing that the 'missing link' that distinguishes *Homo sapiens* from other animals is our remarkable brain size. They believe this is only possible due to community development near rivers, seas and oceans resulting in the significant levels of omega-3 in our diet necessary to build such large brains. The marine environment is our main source of these essential omega-3s, i.e. fish, fish oils and cod liver oil.

Epidemiological research also shows us that peoples existing on a high-fish diet suffer less heart and arthritic disease.

One example: The Faroe Islands are situated in the North Atlantic between Scotland, Iceland and Norway. Abundant fishing grounds supply the Faroese with a major part of their diet. In 1988, a team of medical researchers recorded that the incidence of rheumatoid arthritis was much lower here than in other parts of the world. The 1 per cent of the population it did affect suffered only a mild form of the disease and 90 per cent of these remained able-bodied and 50 per cent still worked full-time. It was concluded that their fishy diet protected the Islanders.

Studies of other populations have identified that fish-eating peoples like the Greenland Inuits and the coastal Japanese are protected against inflammatory and heart disease.

John E. Croft has a book of his own. The title – *Natural Relief from Arthritis* – states a commendable goal. I agree with him on one major point. There is great truth in his concluding comments. He writes:

So far, using substances found on land, we have not been successful in finding a cure for diseases like cancer, leukemia and multiple sclerosis. The treatments which remedy these and other serious disorders may very well be awaiting discovery in a very obvious place – the ocean.

End quote. A perfect summary. No wonder I am such a staunch advocate of cod liver oil.

Chapter IV
Absorb The Oils:
It Can Be Done!

From the very start I have always maintained that certain oils contained in certain foods can be beneficial to the linings of your joints.

I've been saying this for 30 years. The human body is capable of digesting and absorbing oils. It can self-lubricate arthritic joints.

By eliminating dryness, your joints can move more easily, pain recedes, and better health is the happy reward.

This theory of 'lubrication' which I advanced was immediately challenged by some segments of the medical profession. The critics, doctors among them, made statements like these: 'The dietary plan proposed by Alexander is too simple an answer. He's a layman, so he probably knows very little about basic physiology.'

Apparently they would prefer that I use more 'medical language' and more technical terms. Whenever I discuss human anatomy or digestive organs, I guess they want me to sound like a doctor. Why? Just to prove I have education and knowledge on these topics?

My first responsibility is to you, the reader. I will not subject you to a complicated vocabulary. My message can be told in clear, understandable words.

Imagine that you are looking at the interior of your small intestine . . . Inside your gastro-intestinal tract are thousands of tiny projections, each called a villus. Inside each one are capillaries which house 'lacteals' – the lymph vessels that can help carry the proper dietary oils to arthritic joints. Your primary goal should be to deliver Vitamin D3 oil (cholecalciferol) to the lacteals.

This route I am describing is using systemic circulation to carry oil globules, microscopically small, toward the lining of your joints.

For example, when the cod liver oil mixture which I recommend is taken on an empty stomach, it is carried by the lacteals until it is later absorbed or assimilated within the body.

These lymph vessels (the lacteals) then transport the oil to a major oil collecting 'depot' within your system known as the cisterna chyli. Then it is picked up by the thoracic duct – and the cod liver oil is delivered into the lymphatic system. It is piped into the main bloodstream as minute chylomicrons.

By taking cod liver oil you are 'loading' the chylomicrons with Vitamin D, Vitamin A, and Vitamin F.

You are using systemic circulation to carry these oil-soluble

> As previously detailed, Vitamin F is no longer used as a term for the essential fatty acids.

vitamins and essential fatty acids to the locations in your body where they are needed most.

In effect, when you bypass the greedy liver in this manner, you can deliver Vitamin D intact to the lining of the joints!

This process of absorbing the oils works best when you don't drink water with your meals. If you omit water, I maintain that your digestive system can deliver approximately 90 per cent of the Vitamin D oil to your lacteals. The capillaries will capture the remaining 10 per cent. But, healthwise, you're way ahead.

I insist that oil can 'travel' to the linings of your joints. Some doctors have questioned this fact which baffles me, because this is not just my theory. It is not something I invented. Many distinguished scientists did the initial research. They deserve full credit for exploring this type of lipid metabolism.

We are discussing how oil is metabolized – how it is absorbed by your body. Medical literature has been publishing learned articles on this topic for the past 40 years!

Source Material: Proof About 'Absorbing' Oils

The real pioneer in this field of lipid (oil) metabolism is Dr. A.C. Frazer. Way back in 1945, he reported the results of his research in *The Journal of Physiology*.

Dr. Frazer conducted tests which showed how hydrolyzed oils can be drawn primarily into the lymphatic system of your body. Instead of traveling the portal route – to your liver – these long-chain fatty acids would be absorbed by the lymph ducts.

In my first book, 33 years ago, I mentioned Dr. Frazer's work. I also commended Dr. Abraham White, the noted biochemist at Yale University. He wrote a revealing chapter on this subject. It appeared in a book entitled *Diseases of the Metabolism*. That volume was published in 1947.

I repeat, this theory is not new . . . and it is not revolutionary.

Both of these men inspired my thinking . . . set me off on a search for more answers.

For example, one factor which I learned from Dr. Frazer was the importance of using hydrolyzed oil. Break down the oil globules – emulsify them, so they can travel through your digestive system more easily. That's why I recommend that you mix cod liver oil with orange juice or milk. Shake it well to make the emulsification more complete.

For my comments on milk and a further 'cod liver oil cocktail' suggestion, turn to page 103.

As the years went by, the evidence mounted. In 1959, Dr. Samuel Gurin contributed his findings to the fourth edition of *Diseases of the Metabolism*. He told how investigations were conducted concerning the route of transport of saturated acids with different chain lengths.

Let me clarify what 'chain length' means. It is simply a term that biochemists use to describe the carbon content in various fatty acids. For instance, cod liver oil is considered to be 'long chain', because it contains 22 atoms of carbon per molecule.

Dale Alexander is getting much closer to the truth here. But it would have been more precise to describe cod liver oil as 'containing long-chain polyunsaturated fatty acids (LCPs)'. Both EPA and DHA are LCPs. In fact EPA has 20 carbon atoms with five double bonds (20:5) and DHA has 22 carbon atoms with six double bonds (22:6).

Butter and eggs are in the 'short chain' category, with only about four carbon atoms in their molecular structure.

Dr. Gurin cited research work which suggested that the shorter chain acids may be transported largely by way of the portal circulation. In other words, through the liver!

But, to quote Dr. Gurin: 'It would appear, therefore, that the long-chain saturated and unsaturated acids are <u>preferentially transported</u> by way of the <u>lymphatic</u> system.'

The underlining is mine, for emphasis. He is stating, as I have for years, the same basic fact: Oils can travel through your body via lymph ducts.

When I learned it was possible to 'direct' the flow of oils to various parts of one's body, that fact became the cornerstone for my future research.

At that time – in the early 1940s – there was one major question still unresolved. Some way, I had to determine which oil would be most beneficial for arthritics.

By poring over medical journals, for weeks on end, I discovered repeated references to cod liver oil. You already know, from Chapter III, how medical history favored this oil. It was the logical choice.

Dietary common sense was all I prescribed in my original book. My nutritional findings are not based on some mysterious formula. Any pre-med student who is taught basic physiology will realize how metabolism works. Even so, some doctors still act surprised when my dietary program reduces pain.

The key element to be metabolized by your body is cod liver oil. Mainly because this substance contains Vitamin D_3 for the lubrication process.

Cod liver oil is an excellent nutritional supplement and an outstanding natural treatment for the pain and stiffness of arthritis. However, science tells us that the key elements to be metabolized by your body are the omega-3 fatty acids IN cod liver oil.

It is the omega-3s that are responsible for arthritis relief.

Vitamin D is both a vitamin and a hormone. It is undoubtedly necessary for good health and essential for bone growth and continuing bone health, but it is not quite as active as Dale Alexander describes. There are many reasons why Vitamin D was thought to affect the cure: without good supplies of Vitamin D, calcium will not be efficiently laid down as bone, resulting in the deficiency disease, rickets. Symptoms of rickets include aching of the legs, knees and other joints. There may also be tender swelling of ankle and wrist joints, swelling at the ends of long bones and vulnerability to infections. In adults, lack of Vitamin D results in a condition known as osteomalacia, where the bone is remade without adequate calcium salts. Bones become weakened and early symptoms are vague aches and pains in the bones which may well be described as arthritis or rheumatism.

Vitamin D is made by the action of sunlight on the skin and is also found in foods such as egg yolks, butter, cheese and fortified margarines. Vitamin D is the variant found in fatty fish and cod liver oil.

If you are ready to try a nutritional approach, study mine. Compare my plan with other diets – a rash of them are being announced on newsstands.

Every few weeks, another national magazine will suddenly feature a major story on what happens when arthritics seek relief through some form of diet.

Prevention Magazine: Publishing The Truth!

Arthritis was the subject of a five-page article in *Prevention* magazine not long ago. I congratulate the editors and staff of that publication for a superb job of reporting.

Everyone afflicted with arthritis could relate to what the writer said. He gave an honest, up-to-date description of the latest methods which arthritics are using to gain relief.

I was so favorably impressed, I telephoned the magazine. My purpose was to commend the staff; they did some outstanding research work, compiling background facts for the article.

An editorial decision was made at *Prevention* which caused the magazine to conduct an entire project on arthritis. In one edition, the editor, Robert Rodale, invited his loyal readers who had arthritis to send him letters. He asked for a progress report on what steps they were taking to fight the disease.

The mail response was immediate, and overwhelming!

Hundreds of letters poured into *Prevention*'s offices. Some were tragic, as arthritics told their own stories of pain and anguish.

But many of the letters offered hope, talked of remedies which had worked successfully. People wanted to share their experiences in order to help arthritics everywhere. So Editor Rodale wrote a special column based on his incoming mail. (I shall quote from that remarkable column later in this chapter.)

I am especially pleased that this authentic survey was conducted, and by this unique publication, because I have watched the growth of *Prevention* since it was founded back in 1949. When it was still a small magazine, I was lecturing in Allentown, Pennsylvania. Jerome Rodale invited me to his home, to have dinner. We sat around and talked about his dreams to publish an important magazine to serve the health-conscious public.

Even then, in 1952, in regard to arthritis I was a proponent of proper diet and cod liver oil. I told Jerome Rodale about my theories. On many subjects, he and I were of the same mind. We believed that people should have civil liberty, freedom of choice in matters of personal health, as long as such choices do not infringe upon the liberties of others.

Robert Rodale became Editor, and often stated courageous views on many health topics, carrying on the tradition of his father.

Here is an example of editorial bravery. Robert Rodale devoted his entire column to various methods whereby his readers who suffer from arthritis could achieve alternative pain relief. He wrote:

Perhaps some day no one will be surprised or put off by anecdotal information. And maybe no one will raise an eyebrow when they hear of the alternative arthritis therapies you detail in your letters. Massages, hot baths or showers, ice packs, heating pads, positive visualization (imagining a reduction in pain), alfalfa tablets, acupuncture – many of you swear by these and others. Some are known painkillers, others make good physiological sense though there's little or no research yet to confirm them, and a few are just plain mysterious. They all, however, fall under the grand principle that so many arthritis victims have come to respect: If it relieves the hurt, it's good medicine.

Unlike Dale Alexander, I came to health and nutrition from a preventive medicine background. Now I know that this can be a distinct advantage. Although nutrition for health protection and disease prevention is at last beginning to achieve the status and emphasis it warrants (increased fruit and vegetable consumption and saturated fat reduction are two welcome examples), even now, mainstream medicine has a narrow focus on 'curing' disease with surgery or drugs. Nutritional and 'constitutional' solutions are still viewed with suspicion, and therapeutic claims for them are largely dismissed. Dale Alexander was widely criticized in his time. The overwhelming reason is that very few of these 'therapies' have undergone, or could undergo, the 'double-blind placebo'* trials demanded for new drugs.

I fully understand, and would insist, that powerful drugs must be fully tested before being approved for therapeutic use. However, when pharmaceutical companies and physicians ignore or, worse, denigrate non-drug or 'alternative' remedies because they have not

*Double-blind placebo trials are conducted using two groups. One group is given the drug being tested, the other is given a dummy. Neither the people in the groups nor the researchers tracking the results know which is which.

undergone stringent trials, I see red! When medicine has proved either ineffectual or produces side effects that are possibly worse than the condition they are supposed to treat, how can the profession pour scorn on something because it is supported only by strong 'anecdotal evidence' (people say it works!). If a product, special diet or other non-drug therapy makes patients feel better, relieves their pain and allows them to resume tasks they were previously unable to tackle, surely that has a value? Cod liver oil is safe and its only side-effects are improved hair, skin and nail condition.

To my way of thinking, 'anecdotal evidence' is an impressive measure of performance and this is where cod liver oil scores so highly. Thousands of arthritis sufferers all over the world swear that cod liver oil has helped relieve their symptoms.

The trials that have been conducted to date using cod liver oil have produced a range of proven benefits, and several more are in the pipeline. But if it works for you as it did for me, for Dale Alexander's mother and the thousands both he and I have met over the years, then I'm sure you don't need to wait for further proof! You have nothing to lose!

One alternative remedy that wears that label more than most is cod liver oil. In our informal poll it drew an extraordinary amount of praise, and I think I know why. A while back some researchers at Brusch Medical Center in Cambridge, Massachusetts, gave daily doses of the supplement to nearly a hundred arthritics (some suffering from osteoarthritis, others from rheumatoid arthritis, others with gout). The result was a major improvement in 93 per cent of the patients. They had less fatigue, less swelling and better mobility. And these people had failed just about every conventional arthritis treatment you can name.

Here's a typical assessment of cod liver oil's effect on arthritis symptoms:

> My osteoarthritis frightened me most when it began to spread. First it struck my hands, then one knee stiffened, then the other. I couldn't sit unless my right leg was extended and supported. Then suddenly my left knee became much more inflamed and tender. I feared that I was losing my ability to walk. But about that time I heard about cod liver oil for arthritis. So I started taking a tablespoon of it just before bedtime, and very quickly my most painful symptoms eased up. Now I can actually do my gardening again.*

*Author's note: That letter, from a reader of *Prevention* magazine who lived in Rochester, New York, is very similar to the mail I receive from people who have studied my previous book. After they add cod liver oil to their daily diet, they report definite results.

I would also like to make one other observation, just as an historic footnote. This magazine article quoted above mentions the research work performed at the Brusch Medical Center. I am pleased to say that it was I who initiated that series of tests years ago. I requested that clinical evaluation of my theories. The patients followed my dietary rules and were given cod liver oil. Some members of the medical profession have discounted and disparaged the Brusch experiments, but I still maintain that it was a valuable research project.

By changing their sequence of eating, some of those patients had a beneficial drop in their cholesterol levels – by as much as 30 per cent. Also, abnormal levels of blood sugar dropped to normal ranges.

'Maybe the oil's secret is its high content of Vitamin D,

the nutrient that helps keep your body using its calcium.

> See my earlier comments on the value of Vitamin D.

Or maybe the active ingredient is some unknown substance that enhances joint lubrication.

> Undiscovered then but now known to be the omega-3s that damp down inflammation to achieve a similar end result — pain relief and restored mobility.

Whatever the biochemistry is, you can be sure that to those in pain, relief itself counts far more than its cause.

And I suspect that in the long run, the specific remedy isn't nearly as important as the attitudes that engender it. The courage to never give any ground to the pain, the good sense to stay open to healing options – this is the right stuff. And plenty of you have it.'

To those inspiring statements by the Editor of *Prevention* magazine, I can only add one word: 'Amen!'

Doctors Denounce Diet – They Offer 'Aspirin' Instead!

They are still doing it, almost every physician in practice today. To treat arthritis, they usually prescribe some pain killer, available at your local pharmacy.

Drugs are the most popular antidote. As students in medical school, fledgling doctors were taught to rely on pharmaceutical products. Courses were given on which 'pills' were best. They learned about all the medicaments being manufactured – one for every disease in the book!

Unfortunately, in most cases, they had a great gap in their education. Very few classes were held on nutrition.

They graduated, with their M.D. degrees. But most members of the medical profession still have a 'blind spot' concerning proper diet.

> Nutrition, regrettably, still forms only a small part of a medical student's syllabus – in the US, 99 out of 127 medical schools have no nutrition class offerings – but pressure from 'below' – ordinary people like you and me who do not want to feed their body with a cocktail of chemicals – is slowly changing attitudes. In the case of arthritis this is particularly true as there is as yet no drug that can help everyone – without side-effects.

However, let's be fair. Let's consider 'drugs', and evaluate some actual products, old and new, which have been prescribed for arthritics.

To cover this topic, truthfully, follows an entire chapter about drugs. Read on . . .

Chapter V

Drugs To Relieve Arthritis: Just A Dream?

Throughout history real doctors and witch doctors have been sticking needles into people, using drugs to 'cure' arthritis.

Sometimes their use of injections has been based on nothing more than wishful thinking. The ancient Chinese, for example, were treated with a golden needle. If the joints in their shoulders ached, they would show their doctor the exact spot. Then he stuck the patient with a needle – containing no serum or vaccine – just the needle! (This may have been the prelude to the healing art now known as acupuncture.)

In the sixteenth century, some medicine men in France began to prescribe 'gold salts' to relieve arthritic pains. Porterius, a French physician, started using colloidal gold compounds – and certain doctors still recommend this metallic substance to this very day.

A study reported in 1997 found that a joint on the ring finger of a woman's left hand had been spared the rheumatoid arthritis erosion seen in the other joints of both her hands. Aware of the fact that gold had been used as a drug in the treatment of rheumatic problems since the turn of the century, the investigators speculated that 'gold molecules from her rings may have passed through the skin', accumulated in the joint and slowed disease progression in that area. Follow-up studies revealed that

ring-wearers had up to three times 'less articular erosion'
in the knuckle joint nearest the ring compared with joints
on other fingers. However, there could be other reasons
for the difference, such as the fact that the left hand is
normally less used than the right. Another factor to be
taken into consideration is that severe arthritis leads to
such swelling of the joints that the wearing of rings has to
be abandoned altogether. If these people were compared
to ring-wearers, a false conclusion could be reached. As
gold is known to have positive effects on cellular and bone
immune response, further trials are merited.

The point I am making is that no injection has yet been
discovered which can stop the worldwide spread of arthritis.
Drugs have not prevented the tragic growth of this disease. No
pills can conquer arthritis. The pharmaceutical companies are
still searching for the answer.

There are too many types of arthritic ailments – too many
categories of pain – for any one drug to be totally effective.

I do not deny that medical science has tried to find a potent
product for drug therapy. Many readers of this book are
probably ingesting pills or taking injections because someone
told them they might help to some degree.

The mainstays of arthritis relief today are the non-
steroidal anti-inflammatory drugs (NSAIDs). Treatment
for osteoarthritis is virtually limited to analgesics for pain
relief, with NSAIDs used intermittently for patients
whose symptoms vary. According to a report from the
Arthritis and Rheumatism Council, however, 'Most
interventions are untested, reflecting the difficulty of
doing long-term clinical studies in a complex variable

condition. Clinical management must be based on being logical and not doing harm.'

The analgesic paracetamol can improve pain and tenderness and give some functional improvement, but paracetamol overdose is dangerous as it can cause liver damage. For this reason, the dosage cannot be stepped up when breakthrough pain occurs.

NSAIDs in low dosage act as painkillers while higher doses have an anti-inflammatory action. NSAIDs inhibit the production of pro-inflammatory prostaglandins (as do the omega-3s in cod liver oil). However, after 2-3 weeks the use of NSAIDs actually causes increased inflammation. Figures reveal that only 60 per cent of patients will respond to any particular NSAID although they may gain benefit if switched to another. A paper published in the *Drugs and Therapeutics Bulletin* in 1994 stated that 'The potential benefits of treatment with an NSAID must be weighed against the risks, and alternative treatment should always be considered'. The risks are considerable:

* In the elderly there is a risk of serious side-effects, even fatalities.
* May cause deterioration of kidney function in those with kidney, heart or liver problems.
* May cause one or more of the following side-effects: nausea, diarrhoea, indigestion, bleeding and ulceration, headache, vertigo, tinnitus, light sensitivity and blood in the urine.
* Have been known to cause kidney failure, liver damage, rare lung problems, pancreatitis and aseptic meningitis.

The list of arthritics for whom doctors would not be

prepared to prescribe NSAIDs include patients who:

* Have a peptic ulcer
* Have a history of hypersensitivity
* Are pregnant or breastfeeding
* Suffer from an allergic disorder caused or made worse by any NSAID
* Have a blood clotting disorder

Research into NSAIDs has produced positive evidence in favor of fish oil supplements. In four trials, fish oil supplements helped to relieve joint tenderness and fatigue and in the latter three enabled a reduction in the dose of NSAIDs. The relationship between dietary supplementation with cod liver oil and the intensity of pain in people with musculoskeletal pain found that taking cod liver oil seemed to reduce pain overall. It has also been found that taking cod liver oil with NSAIDs can reduce the incidence of gatrointestinal side-effects. Most trials into fish oils alone report a decrease in morning stiffness, swelling, the number of painful joints and all over pain.

The favorites, for oral consumption, now include everything from aspirin, to colchicine for gouty arthritis, to phenylbutazone for rheumatoid illness.

When Dale Alexander wrote so dismissively about aspirin, its only value was as a painkiller. Aspirin's role as an anti-inflammatory agent and anticoagulant is a more recent discovery. One of the group of NSAIDs, its mode of action is similar to that of the omega-3s – it interferes with the production of certain prostaglandins that promote inflammation and platelet aggregation. However, aspirin does have undesirable side-effects. It can cause stomach inflammation and irritate the gut lining so that some molecules can pass through the gut wall into the bloodstream and increase the risk of food intolerance. Aspirin can also make some inflammatory conditions worse, notably asthma for people who are both aspirin-sensitive and asthmatic.

What Happened To Cortisone?

Synthetic cortisone, taken orally or by injection, has started to fade from the limelight. It has lost its appeal among many doctors and patients.

The decline began in about 1965. By then, too many victims of arthritis were reporting harmful side-effects from using test-tube cortisone. While the drug did bring temporary pain relief to some people, this gain was often nullified when they developed several other annoying afflictions.

Patients learned that synthetic cortisone had a 'ballooning' effect on their faces. In addition to becoming 'moon-faced', some people began to grow hair in the wrong places, like women suddenly finding they had mustaches.

Worse, many women who were in their menopausal stage discovered that the cortisone drug would cause accentuated flushing and high blood pressure. Cortisone also has a nasty habit – after 2 or 3 injections into the same area – of starting to break down the connective tissues that support the joint area, including the joint capsule.

I am not clairvoyant. But even 35 years ago I was urging arthritics to manufacture their own natural cortisone.

Yes, within your body, right now, cortisone is being secreted from the outer 'bark' or layers of your adrenal glands. And this natural cortisone is of a higher quality than any concocted version you can find in a pharmacy.

The secret is, of course, to stimulate your adrenal glands. Activate the adrenals, so they create more and better cortisone.

It has been proven that the adrenals will respond to a steroid, like Vitamin D. Use cod liver oil as the stimulator. Mix the oil with orange juice, as described in this book. If you emulsify the cod liver oil, you can send oil bubbles containing the nutritive Vitamin D to your adrenal glands. Simple and safe. You will not experience any harmful side-effects.

Cortisone, made the natural way, has a heavier quality. It is more 'sticky' and may increase the consistency of the collagen in your body.

(Collagen is that glue-like protein substance which supports bone, cartilage, ligaments, tendons and other connective tissues.)

To sum it up, I am in favor of cortisone if you allow nature to make it for you. When you create it internally you add viscosity to your collagen – so that oils will be held in place near your joints.

In a way, what we are talking about in this chapter is drug abuse. Too many drugs prescribed for arthritics are causing abusive side-effects, harmful to your body. Dr. Robert Mendelsohn cited a sad example . . . so typical and truthful that I have quoted his remarks. (See pages 174–5 of this book.)

A Drug Worth Mentioning: DMSO

It may be the most talked about drug in the world today. A full-scale controversy is raging, and I certainly intend to offer my opinions on the value of DMSO.

Dimethyl Sulfoxide (which the public knows as DMSO) has already survived intense criticism, and has earned our serious consideration as a weapon against arthritis.

DMSO may be the only drug to receive favorable mention in this entire book. I am inclined to admit that this natural product does bring temporary relief for some types of arthritis. I'll be more specific in just a moment. But, first, let's examine the pro and con arguments which have made DMSO hard to purchase anywhere in the United States.

Arthritics are running off to Mexico, paying 'rip-off' prices to remote clinics, in order to obtain injections of DMSO.

The Federal Drug Administration, and other governmental agencies in the United States, have been dead set against DMSO – blocking its sale as a prescriptive drug.

While the fight over DMSO will soon be making headline news in print, it was actually television that fueled the fires and stirred up nationwide debate. *60 Minutes* – the top-rated news program on CBS television – did a special report on DMSO.

Mike Wallace interviewed Dr. Stanley Jacob, the leading spokesman for DMSO. The therapeutical effects of the drug were first discovered by Dr. Jacob in 1963. He and his associate – Robert Herschler, an organic chemist – did their research work in Oregon.

DMSO is derived from a substance which is found inside trees. It is called lignin, the material nature uses to cement cells together within each tree.

You can apply DMSO topically, which means you just rub it on your skin. Dr. Jacob has proved that DMSO can penetrate the skin, travel through the bloodstream, and cause relief from pain. It works for many patients, people who suffer from a wide variety of injuries and ailments.

My Research On DMSO ...

I wanted to make sure of the facts before I recommended DMSO to any arthritics. First, I contacted the CBS television network. They provided me with a transcript of the *60 Minutes* broadcast. I have studied the script, and Mike Wallace lived up to his reputation. He fired difficult questions at Dr. Jacob, and he also talked with critics who were highly skeptical about DMSO.

Dr. Jacob passed this test with flying colors. Millions of TV viewers who watched that program are now firmly convinced that DMSO has real merit.

I know how Dr. Jacob felt that night. He was on the spot, facing Mike Wallace. I experienced the same type of interview years ago, early in my career as a nutrition theorist. At the time, the program was called *Nightbeat*. Mike Wallace asked Dale Alexander some sharp, revealing questions. It's a form of cross-examination, an event you never forget.

Before writing these pages about DMSO, I decided to contact Dr. Jacob directly, to discuss with him, personally, the current status of his research on the drug. I found Dr. Jacob at the Oregon Health Sciences University in Portland. Here's what he told me:

The battle to achieve medical acceptance for DMSO is being won. Millions of people can now obtain it, legally, as a prescriptive drug – except in the United States.

In other countries around the world, doctors and hospitals have been officially authorized to use this therapeutic substance.

Switzerland has approved DMSO as a prescriptive drug for treating venous problems, and the Swiss also apply it topically (place it on the skin) as a method to relieve bursitis and arthritis.

Germany and Austria utilize DMSO, as a prescriptive drug, against acute and chronic musculoskeletal disorders.

Canada has accredited dimethyl sulfoxide for both topical and intravenous use against scleroderma (otherwise known as system sclerosis, a disease in which the skin and other connective tissues become thicker and harder than normal. It severely affects the skin of the fingers and face and can cause problems in the blood vessels, the digestive tract, the heart, lungs and kidneys).

Great Britain made DMSO prescriptive, together with, for shingles.

I asked Dr. Jacob if there are any signs that DMSO will be certified in the United States. 'Yes,' he replied, 'there are some favorable indications.'

For example, the drug has already been approved for American doctors to use when their patients have interstitial cystitis. (Victims of this illness have a disabling inflammation of the urinary bladder.)

Dr. Jacob is also encouraged because DMSO has been granted further approval whereby it can be employed in the process of freezing blood platelets. These platelets can then be used during blood transfusions and other procedures in American hospitals.

DMSO, derived from wood pulp, was used for years merely as a solvent, a cleanser to remove paints and varnishes. Even today, the product can be manufactured inexpensively, for about four dollars a quart. But its medical use may have priceless benefits.

My main concern, of course, is to determine the value of DMSO in regard to arthritis. This drug may bring temporary relief. Evidence indicates that it is helpful in rejuvenating non-articular membranes. But I doubt whether it can help the joint linings. They still need lubricating oils. If your bodily joints are afflicted with rheumatoid arthritis, don't expect miracles from DMSO.

DMSO may have been around a long time but its concept is still totally strange to the orthodox medical community. It remains a 'fringe' treatment despite being used for years by athletes to help them with painful muscles and joints.
DMSO's mode of action is unlike accepted therapeutic

principles. It is not a drug in the usual sense since a drug treats disease symptoms. It is claimed that DMSO treats altered cellular function or damaged cells by changing and stabilizing the 'water structure' within the cell. Its proponents say it restores function in illnesses like arthritis, an immune system disease, in ways that are difficult to understand without a degree in physics. I have met with people who are convinced that it has helped relieve their symptoms, but it does not have the support – evidence or advocates – enjoyed by cod liver oil.

Still Another Discovery ... The New Vaccine!

The momentous news came as a complete surprise. Even the way it was announced was most unusual. The first reports on this great medical discovery were released in those sensational tabloid newspapers which are found in supermarkets.

Millions of Americans, standing in line at checkout counters to pay for their groceries, saw the newspaper/magazines. Splashed on the cover of each publication were bold headlines: 'MIRACLE VACCINE BEATS ARTHRITIS' . . . you could read all about it in *The Globe*. 'ARTHRITIS VACCINE . . . It could prevent and cure crippling disease said *The Star*.

According to the news stories, 'thanks to a major medical breakthrough just announced by top research scientists' a revolutionary arthritis vaccine was now being developed that would end pain and suffering for millions of arthritics.

Like you, I quickly began reading these feature articles, filled with optimism. If true, this was the biggest news of the century. Both of these dramatic stories quoted sources at the Scripps Clinic and Research Foundation in La Jolla, California. As an institution, there is none better in the world.

Located a few miles from San Diego, the Scripps Clinic is home base for several scientists – some very brilliant microbiologists and immunologists.

By reading the stories carefully, the public could understand some of the facts. The researchers have apparently discovered a way to regulate the immune system with antibodies produced in their laboratory.

The synthetic molecules (known as anti-idiotype antibodies) are able to force the immune system to destroy out-of-control antibodies – the kind that are believed to cause arthritis.

Dr. R.A. Houghten, at Scripps Clinic, reported that eventually one method of controlling antibodies may be to administer an anti-arthritis injection. It would be similar to a 'shot' given for tetanus after that disease strikes a person.

Another expert quoted in the tabloid newspapers was Dr. Richard Lerner. He discussed the work that he and his associates were doing at Scripps. Supposedly, according to the writer for the tabloid newspaper, Dr. Lerner said: 'I feel very excited and confident this new method will rid people of rheumatoid arthritis.'

My Skeptical Reaction

The more I studied these news reports about the new 'arthritis vaccine' it appeared that I should seek out the real story.

I promptly telephoned Dr. Houghten, at Scripps Clinic. He was not a happy man. He told me that the previous stories gave the wrong impression to the general public.

Vaccinations to eliminate arthritis were not 'just around the corner'. The first steps had been taken, successfully, but it may take several years to develop this technique.

When I tried to reach Dr. Lerner by phone, he was refusing to speak with any further writers or reporters. He was so upset with journalists, that he wouldn't talk anymore.

Apparently, the first stories were too optimistic, too soon. To say the least, the 'announcement' of the miraculous vaccine was premature.

> A sorry epitaph to this story is the fact that there is still no vaccine to 'eliminate' arthritis.

I'm still hopeful that Dr. Houghten and Dr. Lerner, or other men like them, can someday develop a 'miracle drug' to eliminate arthritis. But there's still a long road ahead, and the discovery of that wonder drug may not happen in our lifetime.

That's why I shall continue my crusade to find a better answer, through nutrition.

I have been called an 'Apostle of Good Health' – and I do speak fervently, like a man with a cause. During my lectures, I am apt to become enthusiastic. Some people say that I often sound like a preaching evangelist. If that be the case, let me quote the Bible.

These words (from Isaiah 1v 2) are the truth: 'Hearken diligently unto me and eat ye that which is good.'

Like a missionary with a message, I shall continue to preach the doctrine of good nutrition.

Chapter VI
The Right Foods To Enjoy —
Take Your Choice

Would you like some good news for a change?

That last chapter — about drugs that offer false hopes — was a little depressing. I suggest we talk about happier subjects. If you like delicious meals and tasty treats, these next few pages will offer you some pleasant surprises.

The diet I propose is permissive, easy to follow. You'll have a wide choice of foods — not a long list of restricted items.

You can still eat many of your favorite dishes. To help you recover from arthritis — through nutrition — the 'cure' should not be worse than the disease. I shall not limit you to a strict diet. You won't have to follow some calorie-counting plan that borders on starvation.

I will ask, however, that you make a few changes in your eating habits. I'll name certain 'oil-bearing' foods that you should try. Which meats and vegetables are best? I'll make specific suggestions . . . so you'll know what to look for at your local supermarket.

To cause arthritis pain to subside takes more than just cod liver oil. Your daily diet must also contribute nutritious elements. Take the first step toward better health, by studying these next pages.

The 'Yes' List: Foods Allowed And Recommended

Arthritics who follow my dietary plan can choose any of the following foods. Select the best. . .

FRUITS
Apples
Bananas
Blackberries
Blueberries
Cantaloupe and Honeydew
melon
Cherries
Figs
Peaches
Pears
Plums
Prunes
Raisins
Raspberries
Strawberries

(Fresh fruit, preferably. If in cans, drain off and discard the syrup. Sugar in juices is detrimental if you have arthritis.)

VEGETABLES
Asparagus
Beans
Beets
Broccoli
Brussels sprouts
Cabbage
Carrots
Cauliflower
Celery
Chard
Corn
Cucumber
Eggplant (aubergine)
Endive
Lettuce
Lima beans
Okra
Onions
Peas
Peppers
Potatoes
Radishes
Spinach
Marrow and squash
String beans
Tomatoes
Zucchini (courgettes)

FISH
Clams
Cod
Crab
Flounder
Halibut
Herring (but kippers and
  bloaters only in moderation)
Lobster
Mackerel

Oysters
Pilchard
Salmon
Sardine
Scallops
Shrimp
Swordfish
Tuna
Trout
Whitefish

MEATS
Chicken
Ham (lean)
Hamburger (lean)
Heart (beef)
Kidney
Lamb chops (lean)
Lamb, leg of (lean)
Liver

Pork (center cut, lean)
Roast beef (lean)
Steak sirloin, porterhouse,
  top round, filet mignon,
  T-bone
Tongue
Turkey
Veal

> Meat and dairy products all contain fatty acids – that pro-
> mote the production of pro-inflammatory prostaglandins.
> They should therefore be omitted for maximum benefit.

DAIRY PRODUCTS
Cheese
  Blue cheese
  Cheddar
  Cottage
  Swiss
Eggs

Milk (full-fat homogenized,
pasteurized)

SEEDS
Flaxseeds
Pumpkin seeds
Wheatgerm

For anyone with arthritis, the foods listed above are the most healthful. Use these pages as a guide. You can enjoy everything from 'A' to 'Z' . . . from apples to zucchini. (See Cooking tips, starting on page 153).

You can see, immediately, that the list includes a wide variety of appetizing foods. I've placed very few limits on your choice of edibles. Because I am a firm believer in one doctrine: Eat well to be well!

As you begin my dietary program, in an effort to be helpful, I shall give you some suggested menus – for breakfast, lunch and dinner. (See Chapter XI.)

Later in this book you'll even find a few of my favorite recipes. That's a bonus for the ladies – and for the male 'gourmet cooks' who like to putter around in the kitchen.

But, seriously, I do want you to follow some basic rules concerning these foods. Don't overcook your foods – microwaving destroys many important enzymes – so I'll describe better methods of food preparation.

Think twice about what you eat and drink.

Realize, for example, that water is a vital nutrient that supplies your body with necessary minerals. But learn *when* to drink water.

> Cod liver oil is a food. It is rich in oil-soluble vitamins (and the omega-3 nutrients).

There I go again . . . praising the effectiveness of cod liver oil. Perhaps you would be convinced and share my enthusiasm for this oil if I show you what 'osmosis' can do for arthritic joints.

We have already studied 'digestion' and the way oils are absorbed. (pages 31–4.) Now, let's see what actually happens inside a joint cavity.

Where 'Osmosis' Occurs Within Your Body

I maintain that cod liver oil, when it reaches the joint lining, known as the synovial membrane, is metabolized by this tissue lining.

Throughout this book, I often refer to viscosity – which is the state of the fluid in any joint cavity. If it is viscous, the fluid is more sticky, adhesive and rope-like.

It generally takes three to six months of daily cod liver oil intake to upgrade the quality of the joint fluid viscosity.

Only then is the joint fluid capable of crossing the semipermeable membrane . . . and this process is known as diffusion.

I am describing the only way that the cartilage can survive in a healthy form. Absence of this kind of oil-augmented nutrition causes the cartilage to shrink. The thinner the cartilage becomes, the more osteoarthritis pain is experienced. Why? Because much of the viscosity has left the joint fluid . . . and the amount of fluid has diminished. So, the bones begin to rub against each other. This friction causes the pain.

> The process outlined by Dale Alexander is not yet fully supported by research. Although osmosis is a fundamental means of movement through a membrane and is involved in any cell metabolism, it cannot work as described. On the other hand, there is no doubt that cod liver oil is helpful in arthritis as thousands of people will happily testify. I would also contend that, although this particular aspect of his approach does not yet enjoy medical endorsement, there are still many mysteries that science cannot resolve. As Dale Alexander's advice has so often achieved the desired results from personal observation and experimentation rather than from scientific study, this may well be another example.

The Primary Reason For Osteoarthritis

I define the problem of osteoarthritis very simply. The joint fluid is losing its viscosity – causing a narrowing of the joint space. The cartilage is also becoming thinner, unable to cushion bones.

Your body can perform miraculous feats. This process of 'osmosis' is one of them. Combine the facts on this page with what you have learned about digestion.

With these facts as a foundation, I proceeded to build my entire nutritional plan.

Success stories, from people who have tried my dietary approach, are most inspiring. I receive mail from arthritics of all ages. Women, men, and even children have gained healthful results.

Parents sometimes write to me. When I learn of any child, crippled with arthritis, I am saddened and angered by the tragedy. For these families, perhaps I can offer a few words of encouragement.

Success Against Juvenile Rheumatoid Arthritis

I am happy to report that some progress has been made to alleviate arthritis when it strikes children. While writing this book, I consulted with many medical authorities – including a famous pediatrician.

The expert on children's diseases whom I respect most is Lendon N. Smith, M.D., of Portland, Oregon. Among his accomplishments, he served for 25 years at Good Samaritan and Emanuel Hospitals in Portland.

You may have seen Dr. Smith on television. The TV networks hold him in high esteem for the advice he gives on matters of health. One indication of his stature is the fact that he has been a guest on *The Johnny Carson Show* a total of 42 times!

Dr. Smith told me about his years of pediatric practice, back in Oregon. He diagnosed several cases of this illness among young people, and he would then refer these patients to a rheumatologist. As Dr. Smith tells it, that rheumatologist 'used the standard aspirin, anti-inflammatories and often a course of a cortisone drug.'

'All there was to offer,' says Dr. Smith, 'was medicine to relieve pain and physiotherapy to discourage stiffness. After I moved to a nutritional approach to diseases, I was called by parents who wanted a more comprehensive intervention rather than just symptom relief.'

Dr. Smith tried to help the juveniles through a nutritional program. He augmented their diet by providing them with additional amounts of Vitamin C, calcium, magnesium, B complex vitamins, etc. He supplied his patients with Vitamin D and Vitamin A, usually as cod liver oil.

'I made them stop the sugar, the white flour,' Dr. Smith reports. 'I was shoring up their adrenal glands, so the patients could get well more naturally.'

> This would also boost their immune function. Recent studies have shown that a diet high in sugar and refined carbohydrates depresses the ability of the thymus gland (immune system control) and taxes the pancreas.

(Does this plan of action sound familiar? Yes, it is very close to the approach which I have been recommending for 35 years!)

In conclusion, Dr. Smith made this statement: 'The results came slowly, but the attacks of fever and swollen joints appeared less frequently and were less severe.'

What wonderful words those are! 'Swollen joints appeared

less frequently and were less severe.'

Someday soon that kind of improvement can be yours. If you correct your diet and select the foods I recommend on pages 56–7.

To be sure, you should also observe a few rules regarding the beverages you drink. Don't 'dilute' the benefits you gain from good foods by gulping down too many liquids.

Some beverages you can consume, in moderation; others you should avoid.

Think, then drink. My commonsense advice on this topic begins on the next page.

Chapter VII

Coffee, Tea, Soda Pop – What About Allergies?

Millions of Americans are gulping down coffee, cup after cup, almost like addicts.

Millions of families, throughout the British Isles, are quaffing too much tea.

Millions of children, worldwide, are guzzling soda pop at a rate that's insane.

I would be guilty of a glaring omission if I failed to include in this book some urgent warnings about these beverages. So, in this chapter, I shall offer my special comments about these popular drinks.

Actually, I am not going to tell you to stop drinking coffee and tea. On the contrary, I am merely going to suggest some commonsense rules on how and when to enjoy 'a cuppa coffee' or 'a spot of tea'. I'll even report on some alternative liquids. They taste like your favorite brew, yet they are healthy additions to your diet.

Let's examine the leading thirst-quenchers.

Coffee . . . Plain And Decaffeinated

You may continue to drink coffee, even if you have arthritis, as long as you consume it ten minutes before a meal. If taken with this 'time cushion' for your digestive system, then damage is minimal.

By separating your coffee intake from the meal itself, you ensure that the caffeine and other elements in coffee will not cause any drying effect in your body.

Drinking naturally decaffeinated coffee causes less stress to the immune system. Standard decaffeinated coffee beans requires the addition of new chemicals which often cause added toxicity and can adversely affect your liver and kidneys.

For the least harm to your system, if you are an arthritic, I suggest that you drink your coffee black. Heavy use of cream and sugar complicates rheumatoid arthritis specifically, because it causes more rapid deterioration of an already sensitive joint lining.

Another word of caution: If you use a non-dairy product in your coffee, you should realize that this substance is usually about 65 per cent sugar. Avoid all such substitutes.

Perhaps a better plan for coffee-lovers is to try making a switch to a health food product. There are coffee-like substitutes now on the market which are composed primarily of malt and barley. Instead of being made from coffee beans, these are powdered extracts.

Tea Time: A Habit That's Spreading

We all smile about one British tradition. You've heard how, at a certain time each day, Englishmen all stop work to enjoy a cup of tea. (The fact is, they stop several times daily, for tea. Which is no different than Americans, who take a lot of coffee breaks.)

I'm all for this idea. I have savored 'tea and crumpets' during all my trips to Great Britain. The popularity of tea is growing, throughout the world, so let me make a few simple suggestions, some guidelines for arthritics.

You can drink tea, but please do it at the right time. Ideally, that's ten minutes before any meal, or at least four hours after a meal. Remember that tea is a liquid with 'high surface tension' (which affects the ability of fats to emulsify) and it should not be allowed to conflict with the digestion of oil-bearing foods.

The potential problem with tea is most severe in the British Isles, because much of the tea consumed in England is grown in India – and this type, which they import, has a very high concentration of tannic acid.

Tannic acid has a drying effect on the linings of our bodily joints. So, arthritics, be forewarned.

Dry skin is evident among tea-drinkers, resulting in 'crow's feet' near the eyes. I maintain that too much tannic acid is responsible. Black tea is often drunk very strong. That's another complicating factor.

Across the world, in Japan, again we find millions of people drinking tea. But the Japanese prefer a much milder type. They use smaller amounts of green tea, served in tiny cups. And, usually, they drink it without sugar.

> The use of green tea with its powerful antioxidant properties has wonderful applications to bolster the immune system – an important consideration in the arthritic individual.

In the United States, the addiction to tea has started to mushroom. While most Americans use the milder forms of tea, we go overboard in adding sugar. Then, in summer months, we commit a worse sin by dropping ice cubes into the tea! Iced beverages are suicidal.

The cubes, in a glass of iced tea, will definitely hinder the assimilation process. They fight with your dietary oils.

Herbal tea is a better alternative.

Many readers of my previous books have already discovered the advantages of herbal tea. The pleasing taste has converted millions of people to this drink. It has the natural healing power of herbs, with no additives and no preservatives.

You have your choice of flavors – like cinnamon,

peppermint, rose hips, orange blossom, etc.

Instead of sugar, try adding some honey. For sweetening, I've sometimes used a teaspoon of apple or cherry concentrate. Herbal tea has always been available in health food stores. Today, it has become so popular that many supermarkets now stock this product.

A Horror Story: We're Drowning In Soda Pop!

To help you win your war against arthritis I may have to frighten you, scare you into taking action, so you will pay more attention to your daily diet. That's why I'm now going to write a grim and shocking report about carbonated beverages.

You face an enormous threat to your health, if you are hooked on 'soft' drinks. Yes, we are becoming addicts, unable to resist the fizzy liquids. This habit is taking a terrible toll, causing health problems among adults and children.

In 1990, the American Soft Drinks Association stated that the average American consumes 11 cans a day.

Too many people think that the soda pop craze is limited to youngsters. Not so. Even senior citizens are now quenching their thirst by reaching for a can of cola or some other bubbly concoction.

For the older folks, it all seems innocent enough. They are not drinking liquor. They're just enjoying 'soft' drinks.

Well, let me say, most emphatically, there is nothing 'soft' about soda pop. Those bottles and six-packs contain harsh, harmful ingredients. Arthritics, in particular, are courting disaster if they don't avoid carbonated liquids.

I am not alone in my condemnation of carbonated beverages. Many distinguished doctors have publicly denounced these soft drinks. One comprehensive report, surveying several experts, was published in *Let's Live* magazine. They blamed soda pop as a possible cause for sleeplessness, nightmares, behavioral disturbances, indigestion, burning urine, hyperactivity, tooth cavities, and a wide variety of other ailments.

Among the physicians whom the magazine quoted was a highly-skilled allergist, Dr. Marshall Mandell. He was discussing the potential hazards lurking in bottles and cans.

Look at the contents. You have artificial coloring, artificial flavoring, preservatives and sugar.

First of all, you have simple bad nutrition and drainage of health from all that sugar. It comes into the system as empty calories, bringing no nutrients with it. The soda pop actually has to steal from vitamins, minerals and enzymes already in the body in order to metabolize.

Then you have the allergic reactions. People can be sensitive to any of the components – to the cane sugar, the corn sugar, the artificial coloring or artificial flavoring.

We have tested perhaps 150 to 200 children and in many cases found something in soda pop as the cause of an allergic response.

The coloring, for instance, is made from coal tar, and people who are chemically reactive to it can have all kinds of trouble.

We've seen people react with arthritic pains, generalized itching, an attack of asthma, or a migraine. We've seen kids get confused, angry, and go into a bizarre hyperactive state, pushing furniture around, striking their parents and running up and down the hall screaming.

We saw a case where a child could drink one brand of orange soda and nothing happened. But when he drank another brand, it contained a different ingredient that made him wild and uncontrollable.

Continuing his report on actual case histories, the allergist said:

We had another patient who was diagnosed with a 'nervous bladder'. She had to urinate 15 times a day. Her problem was cola beverages and chocolate, and when we got her off those, her condition completely cleared up.

> I agree with Dale Alexander that food and drink laden with chemicals and with a high sugar or sugar substitute content are responsible for many modern ills. It is no coincidence that the rise in consumption of processed foods and fizzy drinks is echoed by a rise in food intolerance and allergy.

I'll have more to say about allergies shortly. But, first, no discussion about drinking would be complete unless we covered the topics of liquor and beer.

Alcoholic beverages, for adults with arthritis, are permissible – providing you take certain precautions. You can enjoy an occasional highball or cocktail. Just be sure to drink it at least ten minutes before eating – not during your meals.

Your goal is to keep that liquor away from your dietary oil while your foods are being digested.

Oddly enough, it is preferable that arthritics should take their drinks straight, or with plain water. Do not 'mix' with carbonated beverages. Even club soda has an acidity rating of 4.7 and causes your digestive system to work harder, slowing the assimilation of your foods.

Beer is bottled with carbonation to make it foam. That gives it bad marks in my book. For good health, please limit your beer drinking as much as possible. At the very least, wait until three hours after mealtime before imbibing.

I have stated my case. If you give up carbonated beverages, you can avoid allergies and many illnesses. Why trade your health for a few fizzy drinks?

Allergies And Their Relation To Arthritis

When a person develops an allergy to one or several specific foods, this reaction is frequently a warning sign of impending arthritis. The allergic condition is usually characterized by symptoms in some or many parts of the body, including the joints and muscles.

Allergic people, especially those with rheumatoid and osteoarthritis, often have problems in their digestive and respiratory tracts as well as their nervous systems. Their symptoms include colitis with constipation, diarrhoea and cramps; asthma with coughing, wheezing and shortness of breath; migraine headaches with nausea and vomiting; and fatigue.

Different combinations of these afflictions are commonly experienced by millions of arthritics because they suffer from bodywide allergy.

Prominent doctors, some of the leading allergists in America and worldwide, are starting to link allergies with arthritis and are attempting to treat both ailments simultaneously.

The present methods of detecting allergies in human beings have been greatly improved and are much more accurate; they have become an exact science. Back in the 1940s, when I began studying health subjects, allergists would 'scratch' or inject test solutions into a patient's arm to cause mosquito bite-like 'wheals' on the skin. The accepted tests were to introduce certain food, dust, pollen or mold extracts into a person, and then look for 'reactions'.

For many people 'having an allergy' means getting the sneezes and sniffles. Another common complaint is the occurrence of red, itching, watery eyes when certain pollens or dandruff (dander) from house pets is in the air. Perhaps you, or someone you know, will experience an allergic affliction – like breaking out with itchy hives. Or you might develop puffy eyelids and lips.

If you contract any such ailment, go to an allergist. Let him inspect the condition and diagnose the cause.

Now, in the 1980s, there is a much more accurate symptom-duplicating allergy-testing technique. A number of progressive allergists are using this new method. It is known as sublingual (under-the-tongue) provocative testing. Allergenic extracts are placed under the tongue. They are very rapidly absorbed into the circulation and reach all parts of the body.

The sites where allergic reactions occur will flare up, and the patient's familiar symptoms will be reproduced – showing exactly how the substance affects each person.

One noted allergist who has used this sublingual procedure very successfully is Marshall Mandell, M.D., the Medical Director of the New England Foundation for Allergic and Environmental Diseases. (The Foundation is located in Norwalk, Connecticut.)

Dr. Mandell has employed the sublingual technique in more than 1,000,000 tests during the past 20 years!

A well-trained allergist can usually trace the cause in complicated cases. When it's from eating tomatoes, or eggs, or fish, or strawberries, many times the cause is easily detected by the patient.

But I want to discuss a much more serious form of internal allergy – the allergic reactions to food and beverages that occur in and around joints. That painful affliction is now sometimes identified as 'allergic arthritis'.

The damage caused when you contantly consume carbonated soft drinks is enormous. I also deplore the harm you do to yourself when you flood your digestive system with sugar, caffeine and tannic acid, by drinking too many glasses of iced tea.

By making nutritional errors like these, you decrease the overall quality of your health. You lower your resistance and become a candidate for allergies to develop.

Worse, by eating too many wrong foods – or too much of the 'right' foods – the nutritional damage and allergic overloading by such foods can pass your body's threshold of tolerance. The result can be allergies in different parts of the body, some of which can be very uncomfortable. An arthritic may experience a local or generalized reaction in and around the joints. Painful inflammation can develop in the surrounding muscle, and severe fatigue can also occur.

Some allergic diseases do seem to produce a brief attack of arthritis, usually during a severe but shortlived allergic reaction. True allergies are serious, potentially dangerous but, fortunately, fairly rare. More common is food intolerance, which is sometimes associated with rheumatoid arthritis. In both cases, avoidance of the cause is the first line of defence. In the case of true allergic arthritis, when attacks can get progressively worse, treatment for the allergy itself will be necessary.

A New Term: Allergic-arthritis

Due to some important scientific pioneering, the term 'allergic-arthritis' has now come into popular usage. This is a general description which is being applied to many common forms of arthritis.

Earlier in this chapter, I mentioned Dr. Mandell. He is the acknowledged expert on these diseases.

In addition to being a physician, Dr. Mandell is a Diplomate of the American Board of Allergy and Immunology. His prestigious credentials also include being a Fellow of the American College of Allergists.

I found myself in agreement with Dr. Mandell on several points when I read about his allergy-based studies of 'Bio-ecologic' disorders. He has often stated in his writings that good nutrition is essential in the fight against arthritis.

Dr. Mandell urges removing the dietary allergens and eliminating or controlling the environmental substances that are causing or flaring up arthritis. And, then, he recommends 'supporting the patient internally by means of superior nutrition.'

Such a plan of action will also make the arthritic person less susceptible to illness in general.

You have learned, in these past few pages, that allergies can be a serious problem for arthritics. If you do become afflicted, you'll have plenty of company. Many celebrities who appear in Hollywood films and on TV have been victims of allergic ailments.

One famous case is covered in the next chapter: the tale of 'The Sports Star and His Chocolate Bars!'

Chapter VIII

Sports Medicine: How You Can Benefit

As I sit at my typewriter, ready to write this chapter, my mind goes forth to a faraway village in the nation of Greece. The nightly newscasts on TV are featuring stories about the citizens of Olympia who are preparing to light that flaming torch which signals the start of the Olympics.

Soon, athletes from around the globe will be competing for gold medals, as we all applaud and share their spirit of national pride.

I am also fascinated by the mental picture of joggers and runners. Thousands of them have volunteered to help carry the Olympic torch, running in relays from Olympia, Greece, all the way to Los Angeles. (Later in this chapter I will have some comments about marathon runners. We can all learn from their experience, because many of them have suffered from aching muscles and damaged knee joints. They also know which foods to consume to gain maximum energy.)

It's no secret. I'm a sports fan. Baseball, football, hockey, you name it – as long as I can sit and watch.

In the course of my travels as a nutrition theorist, I have made many friends in the world of sports. I have known famous athletes and TV sportscasters. I've also been interviewed by leading newspaper columnists whose bylines are featured on the sports pages.

I am very grateful for the time they have spent with me, and for the friendly interest they have shown in my dietary theories. To indicate just some of my activities in the field of athletics, let me quote two newspaper articles by well-known sportswriters. Here are some excerpts from clippings I saved in my scrapbook.

First, there's one from a humorous column written by Jim Murray of *The Los Angeles Times*. Very appropriately, the headline reads 'Some Food For Thought'. The story concerns the New York Yankees. Yogi Berra was having problems, possibly caused by poor diet. So his coach, Casey Stengel, came to the rescue.

Casey called in nutritionist Dan Dale Alexander, a man whose surest diagnostic tool is the handshake. Most doctors peer down the throat or check the eyes. Dale Alexander checks the grip. If the hand is cold, the rest of you soon will be.

Yogi's hands were not only cold, they were scaly. It was like shaking hands with a fish. Yogi had eczema. 'He couldn't grip a bat, his anxious hands itched so.'

Dale Alexander soon saw the trouble. Scattered around the room were empty bottles of chocolate milk. Yogi drank it by the case. The more he drank, the drier his skin became. Pretty soon, not even golf gloves could help at the bat. Yogi was batting .220, and was itchier than a hound dog.

Alexander says he took Yogi off the chocolate and onto cod liver oil. Dale Alexander thinks cod-liver oil can cure anything from the common cold to falling hair, from arthritis, to arteriosclerosis and, probably, the Johnstown flood. In any case, it cured Yogi's batting average. He ended up the season at .296 and not a scratch on him.

The Western diet has changed dramatically over the past 50 years. Today we eat more salt, sugar, saturated fat and processed foods containing all these and some undesirable chemicals besides. Despite all the advice to the contrary, we eat less fruit, vegetables, fish, and fewer simple 'home-cooked' meals. Our diet no longer meets the needs of our bodies. It is estimated that 90 per cent of Western diets are deficient in the omega-3 fatty acids which are necessary for optimum health, so a daily dose of cod liver oil for all ills is not so far-fetched as it might first seem. Certainly, it will help with circulation (cold hands), skin condition (scaly skin), and it has proved effective in combating arthritis and heart disease. The Vitamin A content of cod liver oil would also help anyone keep a healthy head of hair!

Another columnist, very popular in the Chicago area, is Jack Mabley. He told his readers the true story of my work with Ernie Banks, when he was with the Chicago Cubs baseball team. They were playing the Dodgers, in Los Angeles, when the following incident, reported in Mabley's column in *The Chicago Tribune*, occurred:

Dale Alexander, a nutritionist, walked into the Los Angeles Dodgers' clubhouse to see Ernie Banks and shuddered. 'A nutritional disaster,' Alexander exclaimed. 'Chocolate bars everywhere. Athletes should never be permitted near chocolate bars.'

Banks' friend Billy Williams had suggested that Ernie see Alexander about his bum knees. Alexander said Ernie drank too much tea – vats of it, hot or iced. 'Tannin in tea is used to cure leather,' Alexander said. 'That gives you an idea of how powerful its action is on tissue.'

After he got Banks to switch to cod liver oil from tea, Alexander said, his knees were as good as new in 60 days . . .

[When I met columnist Jack Mabley, it was in his office at *The Chicago Tribune*. I was already past 60 years of age, but I was in robust good health, and I was brimming over with enthusiasm.]

. . . Alexander comes on as a bit eccentric, and he has no degree letters after his name. His main credentials are five books on health, one of which, *Arthritis and Common Sense*, led the national best sellers for several weeks.

. . . 'I've got the skin of a baby,' he beamed as he rubbed his cheeks with both hands 'And this hair,' he added, pointing to a monk's ring around his shining dome, 'is all new. I didn't have a hair on my head for 40 years.'

[I then told Jack Mabley my main message. While praising the value of cod liver oil, I also admitted that I can't even stand the smell of the stuff.]

. . . Alexander says it got a bad reputation because it was taken straight, by the spoonful.

His theory is that the body needs lubricating oil, just as an engine does. He says the oil must get into the bloodstream instead of going first though the liver.

The key to sending the natural oil in our foods to the bloodstream is to escort them with oil-bearing liquids during and after eating, he says. Whole milk and soup qualify.

Not qualifying, he says, are skimmed milk, coffee, tea, soft drinks, liquor, wine, and ice cubes.

I can't see any mad rush for milk and soup by lovers of coffee, tea, soft drinks, and booze. But Alexander swears this is the way to better health.

New refining techniques have improved the taste of cod liver oil to such an extent that many people now take their dose quite happily from a spoon. I've even heard that in the Far East people chew cod liver oil capsules as a treat! Even so, cod liver oil is still not to everyone's taste, so you can take it as Dale Alexander recommends, shaken up in milk or orange juice, or mixed with other fruit juices.

Like many people, I bet on the outcome of sports events. I gamble. In fact, this past year I wagered a grand total of five dollars. A friend of mine wanted to bet me $5.00 on a football game. It was the Super Bowl, and he let me choose my favorite team. Okay, I'll admit it. I lost the $5.00 – 'but wait'll next year!'

Speaking of football, let me tell a brief story about a gridiron superstar. Roman Gabriel was making sports page headlines – as quarterback of the Philadelphia Eagles – when this incident began.

Gabriel was having painful problems affecting one of his knees. As he traveled with the team, he read two of my books – including an earlier edition of *Arthritis and Common Sense.* The football star wrote to me personally, and mailed the letter to my publisher. It was forwarded to me because I was on a lecture tour in Canada.

I telephoned Roman Gabriel, and we talked. It happened that I was scheduled to lecture in Philadelphia about three weeks later. We arranged to meet. When I arrived in the City of Brotherly Love, I went out to the football field where the team was practicing. Roman Gabriel asked me many questions about foods, menus, and cod liver oil. He decided to try my dietary program. About three months later he was pain-free, and able to continue his stellar football career!

We are friends to this day. I talked with Roman Gabriel in Phoenix, Arizona, this month. He is now an outstanding quarterback coach, working for George Allen and the Arizona Wranglers, in the new United States Football League.

These last few pages – about professional baseball and football players – could teach the team owners an important lesson.

The giant athletic organizations sign players to multi-million dollar contracts. To protect their roster of stars, the teams have resident physicians, resident surgeons, trainers, therapists, even astrologers and psychiatrists – but never nutritionists!

I am baffled as to why proper diet is not considered a prime requirement to keep athletes healthy.

A vast series of ailments – ranging from tendinitis to hamstring muscles to rheumatic pain – could be avoided. Team managers must pay more attention to what their players eat and drink.

> Dale Alexander's remarks are prophetic. There has been a huge growth in sports nutrition and most successful teams and individual athletes employ or consult a nutritionist. As a plus, because so many people – young people particularly – are influenced by sport, 'eating right' has acquired a status it was previously struggling to achieve.

One Doctor Who Understands: A Pathologist

I was encouraged to read, not long ago, some comments by Thomas J. Bassler, M.D., which indicated his awareness of foods and diet as a means to accomplish better health.

Dr. Bassler is now doing important work in the Department of Pathology at Centinela Hospital in Inglewood, California. He is nationally known for his research among marathon runners, one of the sports which is always highlighted during the Olympics. Dr. Bassler is currently conducting a study involving 159 marathoners. Some of them ran 10 kilometers (6 miles) and others raced 42 kilometers regularly – more than 26 miles!

Naturally, many of the long-distance runners contract muscular and skeletal damage, sometimes to the point where they require 'orthotic' devices to help treat injuries to their heels, feet or knees.

(Here is a simple definition of 'orthotics' . . . It is the science of developing and fitting surgical devices to activate or supplement a weakened limb. In other words, the use of splints, elastic bandages, braces, etc.)

I decided to meet with Dr. Bassler because of something he wrote. It was an excellent article which was published in *Sports Medicine* magazine. He stated, in print: 'Runners with rheumatoid symptoms may benefit from orthotics, however their nutritional needs should not be overlooked.'

Writing for podiatrists – whose patients are faced with articular tissue problems – Dr. Bassler reported on the value of linoleic acid. I agree that this fatty acid (linoleic) is essential for better health. I recommend certain foods as good sources of linoleic acid. That's one reason why you should include fish, beans, whole grains and other vegetables in your diet.

I traveled to Dr. Bassler's hospital to confer with him personally. We discussed the fatty acids that are found in cod liver oil. I indicated to him that these could be superior to linoleic, even more beneficial for marathon runners, to give them freer joint movement.

We discussed what causes long-distance runners to tire out. What are the right foods to make them last longer, with a 'kick' at the finish line?

Linoleic acid is the 'parent' of the omega-6 family of fatty acids that, like the omega-3 family, are essential nutrients. Arachidonic acid is also from the omega-6 family and is metabolized from linoleic acid. Cod liver oil does not contain arachidonic acid but, as I have described earlier, it does contain two important omega-3 fatty acids . The 'parent' of the omega-3 family is linolenic (or alpha-linolenic) acid. Linolenic acid is found in some nuts and seeds, but the metabolic process needed to convert it to more useful omega-3 EPA and DHA is seldom effective. Cod liver oil's value is that it supplies the omega-3s as EPA and DHA. As a result of dietary changes, the average consumption of the omega-6s has more than doubled in the past 50 years while consumption of the omega-3s has fallen. Our intake of these essential fatty acids is no longer in healthy balance.

This is the same Dr. Bassler who has done notable research on the causes of heart disease. He has recent evidence that poor nutrition is a contributing factor in atherosclerosis. Briefly, let me summarize some of his views on ASCVD, the illness known to millions of people as 'hardening of the arteries'.

Mistakes Which Lead To Atherosclerosis

A too rich diet, lack of exercise, and tobacco use: these are three key errors which Dr. Bassler warns against. If you want to ward off hardening of the arteries, read these next few paragraphs carefully.

Dr. Bassler prepared a medical paper, and it was published in the *Annals of the New York Academy of Sciences*. He made this statement: 'The urban diet is suspect because it lacks food 'fiber', unsaturated fats, ascorbic acid, and tocopherols.'

('Tocopherol' is an alcohol having the properties of Vitamin E. It is isolated from wheat germ oil, or can be produced synthetically.)

The medical report went on to discuss the healthy physical condition of the Masai warriors who live in Africa. They travel great distances, herding cattle on foot, and they seldom suffer from the heart diseases which are common among 'civilized' people. The primitive tribesmen eat a natural diet. They are lucky; they have no refined foods.

Autopsies have been performed on these African warriors. Pathologists found that the coronary arteries of the Masai were enlarged, making them less susceptible to atherosclerosis.

Other scientists have conducted tests based on the diet of the Tarahumara ('Flying Feet') Indians of northern Mexico. Since the days of Montezuma and the Aztec empire, they have been known for their marathon running. They jog through the jungles, in the heat of high noon.

In their village, these Indians stage ceremonial runs – and their physical fitness has been attributed to their anti-atherogenic diet. They live in a fertile valley. In the productive soil they grow corn and beans: natural foods. (One nutritional study included 372 Tarahumara Indians, a sizeable sampling of their dietary habits.)

Some 'Heartening' Facts About Eskimos

The sport of dog-sledding is a grueling test of man's strength and stamina. As they race across the Arctic snow, each sled driver faces bitter cold winds, and I marvel at their endurance as I watch them on TV.

I admire the Eskimo people for another reason. They are among the most healthy individuals in the world. For generations, they have not suffered from arthritis. And, to them, atherosclerosis is extremely rare.

I think I know why . . .

Eskimos have always eaten an abundance of fish. Marine fish oils have helped keep them warm and strong.

Their robust good health has been legendary. But, then, some Eskimos began to migrate to Canada to enjoy the 'benefits' of civilization. When they adopted a diet containing refined foods and carbonated soft drinks, they started to suffer from cardiovascular disease and arthritis.

As long as the Eskimos were eating their normal meals, they never had to worry about hardening of the arteries. Because there is a substance in marine fish oil known as EPA. Some scientists report that this fatty acid can help lower cholesterol and triglyceride levels in the blood. I repeat, cod liver oil contains generous amounts of EPA.

During a research study done at the Oregon Health Sciences Center, a doctor placed patients on a fish diet. It produced beneficial chemical changes in their bloodstreams, including a drop in cholesterol levels.

I have read several reports which substantiate these facts. A different group of patients followed their doctor's advice. He changed them from polyunsaturated vegetable oils to cod liver oil. Result: 'The tendency of their platelets to aggregate and adhere to blood vessel walls appears to have been reduced, making it more difficult for blood clots to form.'

Some physicians still question the merits of cod liver oil. They act surprised when I extol the many advantages of this oil. They accuse me of proposing some 'new-fangled plan' to reduce cholesterol. Don't they realize that serious research began 25 years ago?

Way back in October of 1959, the United States Department of the Interior reported the results of some extensive studies which they authorized. Across the nation, it was headline news: 'RESEARCH PROVES VALUE OF FISH BODY OIL IN REDUCING CHOLESTEROL LEVELS.'

The scientific investigations were conducted by the Bureau of Commercial Fisheries, Fish and Wildlife Service, with the cooperation of the Hormel Institute of the University of Minnesota. The news story said:

A 'saturated' fat, such as lard, congeals at low temperatures. An 'unsaturated' fat does not congeal readily. This is the property which permits oil-laden fish to move freely in waters of low temperature.

Bureau research has shown that about half of the body oil of most species of fish is unsaturated and about 10 per cent of it is highly unsaturated. In other words the potential of fish oil in reducing the cholesterol level is approximately three times that of vegetable oils.

The ability of the omega-3 essential fatty acids to protect against heart disease is well proven and impressive. The case for prevention of a second heart attack is particularly strong. You can take your omega-3s for heart protection in the form of oily fish (herring, sardine, salmon, pilchard, mackerel, trout) but the majority of clinical trials have used fish oil supplements, which also have the benefit of convenience and guaranteed omega-3 content. (Depending on where they were caught and the time of year, fish vary in their omega-3 content.) Two fish meals a week or 200mg omega-3 daily in the form of fish or cod liver oil are recommended for heart health. The omega-3s in fish oils prevent blood platelets (the smallest type of blood cell) from sticking together. This helps minimize the risk of a blood clot which, in narrowed coronary arteries, could result in a heart attack. Fish oils also slow the process of atherogenesis (narrowing of arteries by deposits of fat, protein and cholesterol on artery walls); they widen the arteries; they balance HDL (good) and LDL (bad) cholesterol; they lower raised blood pressure; and they prevent cardiac arrhythmia (irregular heartbeat).

Millions of people saw and read that news story. I wish a few more doctors had.

Enough said. I have given you my heartfelt advice on

atherosclerosis. Now, let's return to the topic of athletes, and the wide, wide world of sports.

Doctors Now 'Specialize' In Sports Medicine

There are more than one million sports injuries in the United States each year, 100,000 of them involving children.

To meet this epidemic of accidents, the medical profession has started to train doctors who will be especially skilled to serve these casualties. An official name has been adopted: 'Sports medicine', the science of preventing, treating and rehabilitating sports injuries. So far, so good.

But I want to make a vital suggestion. This time, will organized medicine please make sure that all these new doctors are also taught some basic facts about nutrition.

Proper foods and menus can have a reparative value, as an athlete recovers from torn ligaments. There are ways to combat Achilles' heel or 'tennis elbow' through natural nutrition.

Already the field of sports medicine includes orthopedic surgeons, podiatrists, chiropractors, dentists and psychologists. All I ask is that these learned experts also inquire about the eating habits of each patient.

Some progress is being made, as this chapter has demonstrated. Scientists study the Eskimos, and explore the diets of Indian marathon runners in Mexico. But it is time to expand these efforts. In our search for nutritional knowledge, let's use the facilities of colleges and medical schools, worldwide.

In the title of this chapter, I spoke of 'How You Can Benefit' from sports medicine. The fact is you are already reaping the rewards. Every time a doctor examines the aching joints of an athlete, he is trying to solve problems that are closely related to

arthritis. Discoveries have been made – and more will come –
to aid arthritics.

Meanwhile, let's all follow the careers of our favorite athletes,
for sheer enjoyment. Root for the high school basketball team,
cheer for a college football hero. Play golf. For many of us,
sports can be the best medicine.

As President of the American Fitness Professionals and
Associates, I am well qualified to endorse Dale Alexander's
remarks. Athletes and sportsmen pay a price for pushing
their body to perform ever greater feats of strength, speed
and endurance and from their experience we have learned
a lot about cardiovascular fitness and the maintenance and
repair of joints, bones and muscle. This knowledge can be
adapted to help everyone. I lecture all over America on a
wide range of sport and fitness-related topics, including
the prevention and treatment of injury and nutrition for
performance and health. I also advise on exercise and diet
programs for special groups, including children, pregnant
women and women who have recently given birth, cardiac
patients and people suffering chronic conditions like
arthritis, diabetes and hypertension.

Chapter IX

Avoid Acidity, And Use Vitamins Wisely

A t each of my lectures – when I invite questions from the audience – there are two topics which seem to puzzle many arthritics.

First, they all want to know my attitude toward citrus fruit. Most everyone admits that they drink fruit juices frequently. Is that a good idea?

Second, when victims of arthritis are speaking freely, they often raise questions about the value of taking vitamin pills. I am always asked for my honest opinion regarding vitamin supplements.

No wonder so many people are somewhat confused by these matters. For years the citrus industry has promoted their juices as a great source of Vitamin C. Meanwhile, pharmaceutical companies are constantly introducing newly concocted multi-vitamin capsules.

Perhaps, in this chapter, I can address both of these issues. I shall dispel some myths, separate fact from fiction. I shall now report on why you face potential problems due to citric acids, and how you can gain potential advantages from certain vitamins.

If you have arthritis, don't ignore the dangers of acidity. Take some preventive measures. I urge you to 'keep your pH up!' Let me explain that statement . . .

Chemists and scientists use the letters 'pH' as a symbol to help designate the degree of acidity in a liquid.

They have established that water has a pH of 7. (Approximately 10,000,000 quarts of water contain 1 gram of hydrogen ion 'acid' and, in mathematics, the logarithm of 10,000,000 is 7.) So, when measuring acids in foods or liquids, anything which registers above 7 is alkaline, and below 7 is acid.

From that mid-point of 7, the scale which denotes acidity descends downward. The lower the pH, the more acid in that food or beverage.

Lemon juice has the lowest rating, in terms of acidity. Scientific tests – to determine the acid content and how caustic it is – proved that lemon juice has a very negative pH of 2.29.

Grapefruit juice is nearly as bad, because it registers a pH level of 2.98.

Orange juice is 3.42 and tomato juice has a pH of 4.18.

When you eat or drink too many acidic foods, you force your blood and your digestive system to work extra hard to neutralize those acids. For instance, your body 'borrows' mineral salts from your blood and tissues to counteract the increased acidity.

'Rob' your tissues in this manner, and they can start to degenerate. Result: a prelude to arthritis.

For all these reasons, you should learn your personal 'acidity rating', so you can maintain your pH at a normal level.

A simple measuring device to determine pH is now available at most drugstores. It is an inexpensive kit containing small strips of nitrazine paper. You place a tiny strip, about the size of a matchstick, under your tongue. In just 10 or 15 seconds, the paper changes color – it records the degree of acidity in your saliva. As a rule, any healthy person will register from 6.0 to 7.

Chew More! Your Saliva Can Combat Those Acids!

Nature gave us saliva, as a key element in our digestive system. It can soften and 'dilute' our foods, and help dissipate the acidity in whatever we eat.

> Saliva contains ptyalin, an alkali that partially breaks down food before it reaches the stomach where stomach acids continue the digestive process.

Gulping down your foods is an unhealthy habit. Don't ignore the chewing and salivating process.

In fact, I even recommend citrus fruits as part of your diet, as long as you chew the fruit. Peel a fresh orange, and enjoy eating it! But stop guzzling glassfuls of citric juices. Don't flood your stomach with ice-cold acidic beverages.

In these pages I have spoken harshly about citrus products. I condemn their acid content. I have always said, however, that you can consume limited amounts of orange juice in a beneficial way.

Mixing orange juice with cod liver oil creates a perfect blend of healthful products. This method, combining both substances, I have recommended for more than 30 years!

The orange juice is 'emulsified' with the oil, and both become easily absorbed.

> Tomato juice also works well and I prefer it.

I have never questioned the fact that orange juice is rich in Vitamin C. That's a great advantage, not to be missed.

The time has come, in this book, for a frank discussion about several different vitamins. Here are my very specific comments.

The Truth About Vitamins, For Victims of Arthritis

In medical circles, among many doctors there is an ongoing

debate. Some physicians are not ready to prescribe vitamins for their arthritic patients. Vitamin D is sometimes credited with having a supporting role, but arthritis, as a disease, is not considered to be a vitamin deficiency.

My own attitude toward using vitamins is more favorable, because I contend that arthritis is really a constitutional disorder, affecting your entire body. If you lack certain vitamins, you must correct that deficiency, or you'll hasten the onslaught of arthritic pains.

Rheumatoid arthritics, in particular, need to increase their supply of Vitamins A, C and D. It is my opinion that these three vitamins are most beneficial. They each play an important role in restoring good health. Let's discuss these vitamins, individually.

Vitamin A favorably affects the matrix of the cartilage. It helps the cartilage to absorb proteins and enzymes.

Vitamin C contributes to the manufacture of good collagen. This enhances the tensile strength of cartilage.

Vitamin D helps to regulate the metabolism of calcium and phosphorus – an essential factor in creating strong, healthy bones and teeth.

I suggest that all arthritics, not just rheumatoid victims, augment their meals by taking a few special vitamins.

If you have osteoarthritis, it might be wise to take 1000mg of Vitamin C at breakfast. Plus a good multi-vitamin-mineral supplement.

If you suffer from musculoskeletal ailments, the same rules apply: try 1000mg. of Vitamin C, and a multi-vitamin-mineral supplement. At breakfast, you should also ingest a 400 I.U. capsule of Vitamin E.

Vitamin E acts as an anti-oxidant and prevents oxidation of the fatty acid molecules in your bloodstream.

May I repeat that rheumatoid arthritics face the most severe problem. Their bones and cartilage have already started a 'self-destruction' process. They need vitamins, urgently, to help arrest this condition.

For them, I recommend the daily intake of five key substances:

1000mg Vitamin C
400 I.U. Vitamin E
100mg Vitamin B
50mg Zinc
50mg Manganese

To complement Dale Alexander's advice, which I can neither dismiss nor endorse, I would offer my own list which details the nutrients often lacking in people with rheumatoid or osteoarthritis:

* Zinc
* Magnesium
* Vitamin E
* Folic acid
* Vitamin B6
* Vitamin B5

How I Gain My Vitamins – From Cod Liver Oil!

It should be obvious by now that I never miss a chance to praise cod liver oil. So naturally, you won't be surprised when I say that this oil is a marvelous source of vitamins.

Personally, I rely on cod liver oil to give me generous amounts of Vitamin A and Vitamin D. I have stayed healthy for 30 years because this oil has the ideal balance – the correct mix of Vitamins A and D, to nourish the human body.

Vitamin E is added to offset as fish oil consumption places greater demands on the body's antioxidation resources. Vitamin E is a powerful antioxidant.

May I make a suggestion? When you go shopping for vitamins in a store, always read the labels on each product very carefully. Be conservative in the amounts you purchase. It is possible to overdose your system by taking too many vitamins, too often. Seek the advice of your doctor as to which vitamins you really require to arrest your particular ailment.

If you ingest too much Vitamin A, it can cause adverse reactions, including the loss of your hair.

Too much Vitamin D can have a toxic effect on your kidneys. So pay close attention to your vitamin intake. Use discretion and your own common sense.

Do you suspect that you are suffering from some form of vitamin deficiency? One way to self-diagnose such a condition is to check your own mouth.

If the tip of your tongue is often raw and red, it could be a signal that you need multi-vitamins. Is the edge of your tongue serrated? When repeated teeth imprints appear along the edges of your tongue, you undoubtedly require more B-complex vitamins.

Another reason for checking labels before you buy is that not all cod liver oils are the same. Recent advances in refining technology have made it possible to increase the omega-3 content of the oil to give you more of these anti-inflammatory, cardioprotective fatty acids. Always check the omega-3 levels of the various products before you buy.

A Reason To Smile: Better Teeth!

One of the happy side-effects of taking cod liver oil – still another advantage – is that you will have fewer dental problems.

You can harden the enamel of your teeth, because the Vitamin D in cod liver oil contains phosphorus. This vitamin also causes a favorable reaction on the calcium which is already in your bloodstream. These two biochemicals (phosphorus and calcium) when properly 'oiled' will travel more easily into the arteries of your teeth.

If you lack Vitamin D, the calcium may travel not into your teeth, but to the surface of your bones. This could bring on

> Vitamin D is essential for the conversion of calcium and is certainly necessary for healthy teeth, but also for healthy bones. Abnormal calcification does occur in certain arthritic conditions (ankylosing spondylitis and pseudogout, for example), but it is not as a result of too much calcium in the diet. And although bony outgrowths are seen in cases of osteoarthritis, they are a secondary effect and not responsible for the main symptoms.

osteoarthritis – you could develop bony deposits at the terminal ends of certain joints, like those in your fingers.

The appearance of your teeth and your mouth should be studied frequently. Look in your mirror, as a preventive measure, to detect certain symptoms of arthritis.

Do you have etch marks on your teeth? Is there erosion, and are your gums starting to recede? Beware, whenever you begin to have 'pink toothbrush' – which could be a tell-tale sign of trouble ahead.

If you discover bleeding gums, don't ignore the warning. That problem is often proof that you have a severe dietary deficiency. For instance, you may lack Vitamin C – and that's a necessary nutrient to improve the collagen of the cartilages in your joints.

Some highly-trained doctors and oral surgeons now agree on one fact. Like me, they have recognized the tremendous value of Vitamin C.

Personally, I shall continue to work closely with dentists everywhere, encouraging them to study my dietary theories. I have no quarrel with the dental profession. On the contrary, dentists are showing increased interest in nutrition. Many are now urging their patients to 'watch what they eat!'

TMJ: 'Arthritis' Of The Jawbone

There is one affliction which is growing at an alarming rate. More and more people are becoming victims of TMJ. The initials stand for 'temporomandibular joint', a technical term for aches and pains in your jawbone.

The mandible is that horseshoe-shaped bone in your lower jaw which carries the lower teeth.

While I was being interviewed on a radio program not long ago, a listener telephoned and described exactly how he hurt. He reported these symptoms: At the jawbone near his ear, he felt something, as though another bone were coming down and painfully pressing his jawbone.

I advised him to see his dentist. First, he should be checked out to determine whether he had any dental malocclusion. If the pain persisted, he could be suffering from TMJ.

In my opinion, TMJ is a form of arthritis. It occurs when you have poor articulation of the lower jaw.

Extensive research has been done by Dr. James C. Greenwood, Clinical Professor of Neurosurgery at the Baylor University College of Medicine. He conducted experiments using Vitamin C to combat bone pain. His findings included proof that this vitamin can stimulate the body's natural effort to repair degraded tissues and can encourage collagen formation.

Helpful Advice From A Prominent Dentist

Among the experts I talked with recently, just before writing this book, is Emanuel Cheraskin, M.D., D.M.D., in Birmingham, Alabama. For many years he has been nationally known as both a medical doctor and as a dentist.

Dr. Cheraskin is professor and Chairman of the Department of Oral Medicine at the University of Alabama. He advocates proper nutrition and eating habits to maintain good health. In fact, he has written several books on the importance of vitamins.

While examining the relationship between Vitamin C and arthritis, Dr. Cheraskin cites the work of Dr. B.E. Ingelmark. According to Dr. Ingelmark, the amount of collagen – the principal portion of the white fibers of connective tissue, cartilage, and bone – is directly dependent upon the amount of protein and Vitamin C available.

Cod liver oil will reach every joint that has articular motion, including the jawbone. To combat or to prevent TMJ, a person should try the dietary program outlined in this book.

I wrote these pages concerning teeth and facial problems with one purpose in mind. My goal was to alert all arthritics, to make you aware that proper dental care is of prime importance. Your mouth and teeth can warn you of impending ailments before they spread to other parts of your body.

You should give dental hygiene a high priority in your life. Consult a dentist regularly. Have your teeth cleaned professionally. Tartar or plaque should be removed (these conditions, incidentally, are usually caused by eating improperly or by a calcium imbalance).

A dentist can also detect and analyze any white deposits or lesions on the roof of your mouth. Such early warning signs could be a forecast of cancer.

To conclude this dental discussion, I can offer you a very

pleasant prospect for the future. From now on you will need fewer trips to the dentist – if you follow the menus and dietary rules set forth in this book. You'll have stronger teeth, and fewer cavities! I learn more about teeth each time I meet with Dr. Cheraskin.

Chapter X
Proper Timing: When To Consume Foods And Liquids

L et's assume that you have selected healthful foods, and you are following the recommended menus. You feel content . . . because you are confident that you have a 'balanced' diet.

Sorry. You may be wrong. Many people wreck the 'balance' in their diet – by drinking the wrong liquids at mealtimes. If you consume certain beverages with your meals, you diminish the nutritional value of all your foods.

In this chapter, I won't be repeating my severe criticism of soda pop. You already know how I detest carbonated drinks and acidic juices. Now, I want to discuss some problems related to drinking water. Then, I'll give you good news on the benefits of milk.

Please refer to my comments on milk on page 99–100.

Timing is crucial. There is a proper sequence for eating foods . . . and important rules as to when you should drink liquids. For example, you should never drink a glass of water at mealtime to 'wash down' healthy morsels of food.

You want to gain the maximum 'lubricating' power – from the edible oils contained in that food. Don't congeal those oils, in your stomach, by drinking ice-cubed water. It's an old adage, but it still holds true: Oil and water don't mix!

How can anyone be 'against' ordinary drinking water? I

assure you, I am not anti-water. The truth is, I recommend that you drink two glasses of water every morning, before breakfast.

Water, preferably warm, can serve as a mild laxative and will help flush your kidneys. It also contains minerals and other helpful properties.

My main suggestion is that you drink water when your stomach is empty. Consume this liquid early in the morning, or four hours after dinner, just before you retire at night.

I do not recommend distilled water. But I am in favor of bottled [still] spring water – that's best of all!

For years, many Americans have been brainwashed into thinking that everybody needs 8 glasses of water per day in order to stay healthy. I believe that is sheer nonsense. If you are eating 2,200 calories per day, your body requires 6½ glasses of some kind of fluid. It can come from milk, from soup, from eating an apple or a piece of celery. Fluids are available each day, from many sources.

If you inundate the grass on your front lawn with too much water, the grass becomes waterlogged and dies. Don't 'waterlog' yourself with too many glassfuls of various liquids. It's unnecessary.

Using ice cubes in your beverages is the most grievous mistake anyone can make. Drinking icy liquids with your meals is a common error. During digestion, your dietary oils will quickly congeal . . . their value is literally lost.

During my lectures, I have sometimes compared the human digestive system with the mechanical parts of an automobile . . .

Your family car has three separate compartments. You provide water for the water pump. You supply oil for the oil pump. And you place gasoline in the tank.

At no time do you 'mix' these liquids. Nobody adds water to the gasoline tank or to the compartment meant for oil.

The human machine has only two pumps. First, there's the heart – which pumps blood. And the second vessel is the stomach – which can pump dietary oils to various points throughout your body.

However, the stomach is unable to pump properly if you are drinking water and other oil-free liquids with your meals.

The Importance Of Waiting ... Before You Drink Liquids

After eating a meal, I maintain that a person should fast for approximately four hours before you drink any oil-free liquid.

Give your stomach time to act.

The lacteals and villi in your gastro-intestinal tract must also have adequate time to assimilate your foods.

The idea of allowing your food to be absorbed – before you cram new foods or liquids into your stomach – is not just a Dale Alexander hypothesis. I have substantial evidence, gathered from The Annals of Internal medicine, which supports this theory.

A report published more than 40 years ago addressed this same topic. An article appeared (in April of 1941) giving credence to the habit of post-absorptive fasting. The author was Dr. Irvine Page, who later became world-renowned for his research on cholesterol.

Dr. Page recommended fasting between meals, to help stabilize cholesterol levels. He gained prominence for his work at the Cleveland Clinic. Now retired, Dr. Page lives in Hyannisport, Massachusetts. I telephoned him, recently, and commended him for his pioneering research related to food and proper eating habits.

I might add that I am against 'snack foods' if they are consumed between meals. Give your stomach at least four hours to digest and assimilate a meal. That's my interpretation of post-absorptive fasting.

Milk: Your Most Valuable Ally Among All Liquids

Milk has been called 'the perfect food' – and I agree that it has fine qualities. Each glass of milk gives you calcium, Vitamins A and D, and it even contains a percentage of butter fat.

Because milk itself is an oil-bearing liquid, it is compatible with the assimilation we are trying to achieve inside our bodies.

While being digested, milk is a liquid with low surface tension, able to assist in transporting oil globules. It can help your dietary oils to bypass your liver, so they can be carried more readily to your lymphatic system.

For all these reasons, I now tell arthritics to mix their cod liver oil with milk. This represents a change from the recommendations I made in my first book. I originally suggested that you prepare a daily mixture made with orange juice and cod liver oil. You can still employ that method, but I now offer you the option of using milk, for equally healthful results.

After much research to find an alternative for orange juice, I found that milk had many advantages. (Another factor involved was that too many people were starting to use the wrong kind of orange juice. In recent years, frozen concentrates of orange juice were invented. Unfortunately, some of my readers were taking cans of concentrate from their refrigerators. They would then add water – a real sin! – to make their orange juice.) If you prefer the taste of orange juice to milk, then just make sure that you use fresh fruit, squeezed by hand.

> Milk is *not* the best way ot take cod liver oil. There are three reasons why I think this.
>
> Firstly, Dale wrote his work initially 40 years ago. The dairy of his day did not contain on average 84 different anti biotics, and RBGH (recombent bovine growth hormone).

This increases the risks of all cancers within the human body due to IGF-1 (Interlukin Growth Factor One).

Secondly, most adults lose the ability to digest lactose as they age, which typically leads to gastric bloating, changes in bowel function, mucous production, and allergic-anti-histimine reactions to the protein casein.

Thirdly, dairy products are devoid of essential fatty acids, but they do contain saturated fats, and omega-6 fatty acids that cause the release of Prostaglandin 2: this particular hormone causes an inflammatory response in the body, particularly within the joints.

Of course, cod liver oil's primary function is to deliver n-3 (DHA and EPA) as well as Vitamin D_3 to reduce the inflammation.

A better choice would be almond milk, soya milk for the essential fats or juice: I have found that orange juice, apricot nectar, peach nectar and tomato juice work well.

At times, I have been asked whether drinking milk will lead to a cholesterol problem. My answer is an emphatic 'No!'

We have been subjected to 'a cholesterol scare', a nationwide alarm which is without foundation. In my opinion, some very vocal cardiologists spoke too hastily and they frightened millions of people. 'Take the milk – and the butter and eggs – out of your diet!' This loud warning temporarily revised the eating habits of too many Americans.

Additional research is now causing this trend to be reversed. I hope for a return to normalcy.

Become a milk drinker. If you want to avoid a heart attack, or a stroke, milk can improve the quality of your arteries. You can add more elasticity to your arteries, so they won't 'balloon out' and explode, like a flat tire. Why suffer an aneurysm or a stroke?

For victims of arthritis, may I emphasize that I am

recommending whole milk. Not skim milk, nor chocolate milk, nor canned milk.

> I cannot endorse Dale Alexander's recommendations for the reasons listed earlier in this chapter.

Stay with whole milk, either homogenized or pasteurized.

Timing Tips For 'Night People' And Late Workers

Your occupation may force you to eat your meals at irregular hours. If you work the 'swing shift' at night, you are not in the habit of having breakfast at 7 a.m. or lunch at noon.

Therefore, perhaps I should give some special suggestions, a different timetable for arthritics who do most of their eating at night. When you read the menus in the next chapter, you can substitute hours of your own choice for all three daily meals.

Just remember the principle of post-absorptive fasting. Wait four hours after each meal before you drink water. (Or, you can drink a glass of water ten minutes before any meal. The main requisite is to consume liquids when your stomach is empty, or as near empty as possible.)

Adjust your taking of cod liver oil based on this same 'empty stomach' approach.

Starting today, enjoy eating! In the pages just ahead, you'll find many delicious meals and recipes.

Cod Liver Oil Schedule

Two principal points must work in harmony.

The dietary regimen must serve as insurance to guarantee the benefits to be derived from sustained use of cod liver oil.

Take the cod liver oil mixture daily for six months. Then take it once or twice a week for your lifetime.

Cod Liver Oil Is Your Key Weapon

Cod liver oil and juice

Using a tablespoon and a small jar, you can employ orange juice or other juices as the emulsifier.

One story that broke during 1998 intrigued me. In essence, it vindicated Americans, and other nationalities, who love ketchup on their food. Apparently, concentrated tomato products contain substances called lycopenes that are health protective.

Lycopenes help prevent cellular damage and abnormal cellular growth and therefore protect against many types of cancer. They may also protect heart health. A study examining the role of beta-carotene and lycopene has expanded lycopene's potential benefits to include protection from UV damage.

It is well documented that tomatoes in their fresh, raw state are good sources of antioxidant vitamins. This new research has uncovered results showing that lycopenes – the natural carotenoids responsible for the red colour in tomatoes – are more bioavailable from tomato paste and that cooked tomatoes, eaten with some oil, release much higher levels. Cooking seems to disrupt the cell structure of the tomato making lycopene MORE available.

This discovery led me to experiment with tomato juice and cod liver oil. If the presence of oil could boost the health value of the lycopenes in the juice without affecting cod liver oil's performance, then we had a potent cocktail indeed! The possibility that a tomato juice/cod liver oil combination could also create a palatable, even tasty, way to take a daily dose of cod liver oil did not escape me!

Here's the recipe I came up with:

In a small jar with a lid, place the following ingredients and shake until well mixed (to emulsify the oil):

1 tbs (1 × 15ml spoon) cod liver oil

8 tbs (4 × 15ml spoons) tomato juice

Dash Tabasco or Worcester sauce – to taste

1 × tsp (1 × 5ml spoon) cider vinegar

Some arthritics may find that tomato juice is one of the foods that aggravate their symptoms. If this applies to you, mix the cod liver oil with a natural food source liquid that suits you.

I recommend that you hand-squeeze half an orange to obtain approximately two tablespoons (2 × 15ml spoons) of juice to place into the jar. (You want no pulp to hinder assimilation.)

Now add one tablespoonful (1 × 15ml spoon) of cod liver oil. Shake the mixture, briskly, for five to ten seconds. When it becomes frothy, drink it promptly. Orange concentrates are not to be used, only fresh fruit. Follow the drinking timetable.

Chapter XI
Menus: A Detailed Guide Of Recommended Meals

To recover from arthritis – to get well and stay well – you will need to concentrate and do some planning, menu planning.

You must remember to avoid certain foods and beverages which are highly acidic, but that's only half the battle. It is equally important that you 'balance' your diet, by eating sufficient quantities of good food each day. In other words, you must plan ahead. Make a list of meals for an entire week. You can include a variety of tasty dishes, and still be eating your way toward better health.

For your guidance, I have compiled a dietary schedule based on very wholesome foods. My suggestions for mealtime are easy to follow.

You may be pleasantly surprised by the menus I offer in these next few pages. Eating should always be an enjoyable experience. These meals – recommended for arthritics – will be appealing to your palate. They are flavorsome and nutritious.

Notice that I have designed three complete sets of menus. They are arranged on a day-by-day basis, a typical guide for an entire week. Depending on the type of arthritis which applies to you, and how severe your affliction may be, you can select the correct group of meals. Bon appetit!

People who have identified a link between their symptoms and their diet through a formal elimination diet or their own observation should of course adapt the menus accordingly. Most health food stores and good supermarkets stock a range of alternatives to those foods likely to cause an allergic response or symptoms of food intolerance.

Advances in the science of nutrition force me to disagree with some of the following suggestions. My recommended changes are shown in italics.

Menus For Those With Osteoarthritis

MONDAY

UPON ARISING
7 a.m.   2 glasses of water (preferably warm)
7:10 a.m.   Cod liver oil mixture
7:40 a.m.   Breakfast

BREAKFAST
Whole grain cereal (1 cup)
Bran (2 tbsp.)
Whole milk (with cereal) (4 oz) – *milk substitutes – soy, rice, almond or potato*
Prunes (6 or 8)

LUNCH
Mixed green salad
Omelette
Whole milk (8 oz) – *omit*

DINNER
Green salad

Chicken casserole – *shrimp or seafood*
Whole grain noodles
Fresh fruit cup
Whole milk (8 oz) – *omit*

TUESDAY

UPON ARISING
7 a.m.   2 glasses of water (preferably warm)
7:10 a.m.   Cod liver oil mixture
7:40 a.m.   Breakfast

BREAKFAST
Poached or soft-boiled eggs (2)
Whole wheat toast
Butter (1 pat) – *omit*
Whole milk (8 oz) – *green or herbal tea*

LUNCH
Bran muffin
Butter (1 pat) – *omit*
Cottage cheese soup – *vegetable soup with beans*
Green salad
Whole milk (8 oz) – *omit*

DINNER
Broiled (grilled) steak – *tuna steak*
Small green salad
Toasted Potato Strips (see Recipes)
Carrots and zucchini (courgettes) steamed
Whole milk (8 oz) – *omit*

WEDNESDAY

UPON ARISING
7 a.m.   2 glasses of water (preferably warm)
7:10 a.m.   Cod liver oil mixture
7:40 a.m.   Breakfast

BREAKFAST
Fresh fruit cup
Cheese and parsley omelette – *small herb omelette*
Whole grain toast (1 slice)
Butter and honey – *omit butter*
Whole milk (8 oz) – *green or herbal tea*

LUNCH
Chicken salad – *seafood salad*
Whole grain savory crackers
Sliced peaches or fresh fruit (in season)
Whole milk (8 oz) – *omit*

DINNER
Spinach salad
Vegetarian dinner
Silky's Nutty Fruit Cake (small slice) (see Recipes)
Whole milk (8 oz) – *omit*

THURSDAY

UPON ARISING
7 a.m.   2 glasses of water (preferably warm)
7:10 a.m.   Cod liver oil mixture
7:40 a.m.   Breakfast

BREAKFAST
Cooked rolled oats (1 cup)
Bran (2 tbsp)
Whole milk (2 oz) – *omit*
Prunes (6 or 8)
Whole milk (6 oz)

LUNCH
Poached eggs on toast (2)
Mixed green salad
Whole milk (8 oz) – *vegetable broth*

DINNER
Broiled (grilled) hamburger meat – *tuna or salmon steak*
Baked potato (1 medium)
Brussels sprouts (½ cup)
Whole milk (8 oz) – *omit*

FRIDAY

UPON ARISING
7 a.m.   2 glasses of water (preferably warm)
7:10 a.m.   Cod liver oil mixture
7:40 a.m.   Breakfast

BREAKFAST
Granola cereal (1 cup)
Bran (2 tbsp)
Whole milk (4 oz) – *soy, almond or rice milk*
Berries and plain whole yoghurt – *omit yoghurt*
Whole milk (4 oz) – *omit*

LUNCH
Tuna sandwich on seven-grain bread
Green salad
Whole milk (8 oz) – *vegetable broth*

DINNER
Gazpacho (see Recipes)
Broiled (grilled) halibut and steamed carrots
Fresh fruit cup
Carob cookie
Whole milk (8 oz) – *green or herbal tea*

SATURDAY

UPON ARISING
7 a.m.   2 glasses of water (preferably warm)
7:10 a.m.   Cod liver oil mixture
7:40 a.m.   Breakfast

BREAKFAST
Buckwheat pancakes
Freckled banana and whole yoghurt – *omit yoghurt*
Whole milk (8 oz) – *omit*

LUNCH
Hamburger patty on sesame roll – *prawn salad on sesame roll*
Green salad
Whole milk (8 oz) – *vegetable broth*

DINNER
Chicken casserole with brown rice – *seafood casserole*
Silky's Nutty Fruit Cake (see Recipes) – *fresh fruits*
Whole milk (8 oz) – *green or herbal tea*

SUNDAY

UPON ARISING
7 a.m.   2 glasses of water (preferably warm)
7:10 a.m.   Cod liver oil mixture
7:40 a.m.   Breakfast

BREAKFAST
Choice of fruit
Corn or bran muffins
Lean bacon or ham – *omit*
Eggs (2) – *omit*
Whole milk (8oz) – *green or herbal tea*

LUNCH
Mixed green salad
Corn tortilla with melted Cheddar cheese – *tortilla with beans and salsa*
Whole milk (8 oz) – *green or herbal tea*

DINNER
Oriental vegetables over brown rice
Whole almonds and chicken on top – *salmon on top*
Tapioca pudding (1 cup) – *fruit cup*
Whole milk (8 oz) – *green or herbal tea*

More than a few senior citizens with arthritis have asked me what they should do if they have trouble in chewing. Sometimes they have ill-fitting dentures.

Here's one suggestion: a raw salad can be mixed in a blender with a little milk.

> I recommend a milk substitute, preferably soy, whenever Dale Alexander uses milk as an ingredient.

Add seasoning or salad dressing. Drink your salad slowly.

Cooked vegetables, still firm, can be homogenized in a blender with some milk. Add a bit of seasoning, as desired. As another variation, just by adding more milk, you create a delicious soup.

If your teeth present no problem, then forge ahead happily, and try these menus.

Chew. Mix your saliva with whatever you eat. Chewing your food adds ptyalin for better digestion. Ptyalin in your saliva is an enzyme that converts starch into various dextrins and maltose.

Menus For Those With Rheumatoid Arthritis

MONDAY

UPON ARISING
7 a.m.   2 glasses of water (preferably warm)
7:10 a.m.   Cod liver oil mixture
7:40 a.m.   Breakfast

BREAKFAST
Special Health Drink (See recipe on page 116)
Vitamin supplements (At breakfast time, daily, if you have rheumatoid arthritis, you should also take the vitamin supplements listed.

LUNCH
Cottage cheese (½ cup) — *bean and vegetable soup*
Fresh fruit slices
Date nut bread
Cream cheese (1 tbsp) — *omit*

Whole milk (8 oz) — *omit*

DINNER
Broiled (grilled) lamb chops (2 small) — *salmon, tuna, herring*
Baked yam
Broccoli (½ cup)
Fluffy Rice Pudding (see Recipes)
Whole milk (8 oz) — *green or herbal tea*

TUESDAY
UPON ARISING
7 a.m.   2 glasses of water (preferably warm)
7:10 a.m.   Cod liver oil mixture
7:40 a.m.   Breakfast

BREAKFAST
Special Health Drink (Same as Monday breakfast)
Vitamin supplements (Same as Monday)

LUNCH
Whole grain English muffin (toasted)
Cheddar cheese (1 slice) — *omit*
Melon (¼)
Whole milk (8 oz) — *green or herbal tea*

DINNER
Clear soup (1 cup)
Oriental Vegetable Delight (see Recipes)
Whole milk (8 oz) — *green or herbal tea*

WEDNESDAY

UPON ARISING
7 a.m.   2 glasses of water (preferably warm)

7:10 a.m.   Cod liver oil mixture
7:40 a.m.   Breakfast

BREAKFAST
Special Health Drink
Vitamin supplements

LUNCH
Fresh fruit salad
Bran muffin (1)
Butter (1 pat) – *honey*
Whole milk (8 oz) – *vegetable broth*

DINNER
Tossed green salad – *salmon or tuna steak*
Broiled (grilled) hamburger steak
Baked potato (1 small)
Swiss chard or other dark green leafy vegetable (1 cup)
Carrot Yoghurt Cake (see Recipes) (1 slice) – *carrot cake*
Whole milk (8 oz) – *green or herbal tea*

THURSDAY

UPON ARISING
7 a.m.   2 glasses of water (preferably warm)
7:10 a.m.   Cod liver oil mixture
7:40 a.m.   Breakfast

BREAKFAST
Special Health Drink
Vitamin supplements

LUNCH
Toss and Fluff Spinach Salad (see Recipes)

Hot corn bread
Butter (1 pat) – *honey*
Whole milk (8 oz) – *green or herbal tea*

DINNER
Spinach salad
Baked Chicken Casserole (see Recipes) – *seafood casserole*
Whole grain noodles (½ cup)
String beans (½ cup)
Whole milk (8 oz) – *green or herbal tea*

FRIDAY

UPON ARISING
7 a.m.   2 glasses of water (preferably warm)
7:10 a.m.   Cod liver oil mixture
7:40 a.m.   Breakfast

BREAKFAST
Special Health Drink
Vitamin supplements

LUNCH
Devilled egg sandwich – *salmon sandwich*
Carrot and celery sticks
Corn chips (½ cup)
Slice of pineapple
Whole milk (8 oz) – *green or herbal tea*

DINNER
Mixed green salad
Broiled (grilled) fish or steak – *fish not meat*
Toasted Potato Strips (see Recipes)
Carrots and peas (½ cup)

Silky's Nutty Fruit Cake (small piece) (see Recipes)
Whole milk (8 oz) – *green or herbal tea*

SATURDAY

UPON ARISING
7 a.m.   2 glasses of water (preferably warm)
7:10 a.m.   Cod liver oil mixture
7:40 a.m.   Breakfast

BREAKFAST
Special Health Drink
Vitamin supplements

LUNCH
Cottage Cheese Vegetable Soup (see Recipes) – *vegetable and bean soup*
Hot corn bread (1 square)
Butter (1 pat) – *omit*
Honey (1 tbsp)
Whole milk (8 oz) – *omit*

DINNER
Mixed green salad
Broiled calves' liver or other meat – *tuna, salmon, trout*
Corn on the cob
Carrot Yoghurt Cake (see Recipes) – *carrot cake*
Whole milk (8 oz) – *green or herbal tea*

SUNDAY

UPON ARISING
7 a.m.   2 glasses of water (preferably warm)
7:10 a.m.   Cod liver oil mixture

7:40 a.m.   Breakfast

BREAKFAST
Special Health Drink
Vitamin supplements

LUNCH
Mixed vegetable salad
Corn tortilla topped with cheddar cheese (grill until cheese
melts) — *tortilla with black beans and salsa*
Whole milk (8 oz) — *green or herbal tea*

DINNER
Chicken broth (1 cup) — *vegetable broth*
Broiled chicken — *white fish*
Buckwheat (Kasha) (1 cup)
Brussels sprouts
Carrot Yoghurt Cake (see Recipes) (1 slice) — *carrot cake*
Whole milk (8 oz) — *green or herbal tea*

In the group of menus you have just read, please note that I ask
you to augment these foods by taking vitamin supplements.
(See the list on page 89–90.)

For victims of rheumatoid arthritis, especially, the formula
published below could be most beneficial.

I recommend that you take this drink daily, for at least six
months. This is how you make it:

SPECIAL HEALTH DRINK
1 tsp chia or flaxseed
1 tsp sunflower seeds
6 oz whole milk — *soy or rice milk*

Soak seeds for 15 minutes in:
1 fertile egg
1 tbsp soybean or sunflower oil – *soybean or flaxseed oil*
1 tbsp acidophilus culture
Pinch of sea kelp powder
½ tsp of rosehip powder
I tsp brewer's or torula yeast – *omit*
1 tsp lecithin
1 tsp malted coconut
1 freckled banana

Blend in a blender and drink. It's a complete breakfast!

Following recent outbreaks of salmonella poisoning, raw egg is inadvisable

Menus For Those With Musculoskeletal Arthritis

If you have musculoskeletal problems (tendonitis, myositis, sciatica rheumatism, bursitis, fibrositis, neuritis, shin splints etc.) I recommend the following meals:

MONDAY

UPON ARISING
7 a.m.   2 glasses of water (preferably warm)
7:10 a.m.   Cod liver oil mixture
7:40 a.m.   Breakfast

BREAKFAST
Whole grain cereal (1 cup)
Bran (2 tbsp)

Whole milk (with cereal) (4 oz) – *soy, almond or rice milk*
Prunes (6 or 8)
Whole milk (4 oz) – *omit*

LUNCH
Mixed green salad
Omelette (2 eggs) – *made with egg substitute*
Whole milk (8 oz) – *green or herbal tea*

DINNER
Waldorf salad (apples, celery, nuts, mayonnaise) – *soy mayonnaise*
Leg of lamb (2 slices) – *fish*
Carrots and peas (1 cup)
Tapioca pudding (½ cup) – *fruit cup*
Whole milk (8 oz) – *green or herbal tea*

TUESDAY

UPON ARISING
7 a.m.   2 glasses of water (preferably warm)
7:10 a.m.   Cod liver oil mixture
7:40 a.m.   Breakfast

BREAKFAST
Poached eggs (2) – *egg substitute*
Whole wheat toast (1 slice)
Whole yoghurt (½ cup) – *omit*
Prunes (6)
Whole milk (8 oz) – *green or herbal tea*

LUNCH
Tossed green salad
Grilled cheese sandwich – *not spread with sprouted seeds*

Apple
Whole milk (8 oz) – *green or herb tea*

DINNER
Vegetable soup (6 oz)
Cheese Enchiladas (see Recipes) (2) – *bean enchilada*
Celery and carrot sticks
Brown rice (½ cup)
Whole milk (8 oz) – *green or herbal tea*

WEDNESDAY

UPON ARISING
7 a.m.   2 glasses of water (preferably warm)
7:10 a.m.   Cod liver oil mixture
7:40 a.m.   Breakfast

BREAKFAST
Granola cereal (½ cup)
Raw wheat germ (2 tbsp.)
Plain whole yoghurt (4 oz) – *omit*
Sliced fresh fruit
Whole milk (8 oz) – *green or herb tea*

LUNCH
Mixed green salad
Brisket of beef (1 slice) – *mixed seafood (in soy mayonnaise if desired)*
Cookie (1) – *cup mixed fruits*
Whole milk (8 oz) – *omit*

DINNER
Lima bean soup (½ cup)
Broiled (grilled) calves' liver or steak – *halibut or cod*
Baked yam (1 small)

String beans (½ cup)
Sliced fruit (½ cup)
Whole milk (8 oz) – *green or herbal tea*

THURSDAY

UPON ARISING
7 a.m.   2 glasses of water (preferably warm)
7:10 a.m.   Cod liver oil mixture
7:40 a.m.   Breakfast

BREAKFAST
Special Health Drink (see recipe on page 116)
Vitamin supplements (Listed on pages 89–90)

LUNCH
Tuna sandwich on whole grain bread
Green romaine (Cos) lettuce and tomato
Pear
Whole milk (8 oz) – *green or herbal tea*

DINNER
Green salad with tomato
Roast pork (2 slices) – *baked trout with almonds*
Baked potato (1 small)
Asparagus (4 spears)
Whole yoghurt and strawberries – *1 cup strawberries or other fruit in season*
Whole milk (8 oz) – *green or herbal tea*

FRIDAY

UPON ARISING
7 a.m.   2 glasses of water (preferably warm)

7:10 a.m.   Cod liver oil mixture
7:40 a.m.   Breakfast

BREAKFAST
Whole grain hot cereal
Raw wheat germ (2 tbsp)
Whole milk (on cereal) (2 oz) – *soy, almond, rice milk*
Whole yoghurt and prunes
Whole milk (6 oz) – *green or herbal tea*

LUNCH
Sliced cold meat (ham, pork, or veal) – *tuna salad sandwich*
Tossed green salad
Cookie – *piece fruit*
Whole milk (8 oz) – *green or herbal tea*

DINNER
Shrimp cocktail
Broiled (grilled) lobster
Toasted Potato Strips (see Recipes)
Stewed tomato (½ cup)
Green beans (½ cup)
Silky's Nutty Fruit Cake (see Recipes) (1 slice)
Whole milk (8 oz) – *green or herbal tea*

SATURDAY

UPON ARISING
7 a.m.   2 glasses of water (preferably warm)
7:10 a.m.   Cod liver oil mixture
7:40 a.m.   Breakfast

BREAKFAST
Choice of fresh fruit

Bran or corn muffin and butter — *use honey instead of butter*
Scrambled eggs (2) — *egg substitute*
Lean ham or bacon — *smoked salmon*
Whole milk (8 oz) — *green or herb tea*

LUNCH
Chicken salad — *mixed bean and vegetable salad*
Corn bread (1 square)
Butter (1 pat) — *honey*
Melon (¼)

DINNER
Vegetable soup
Cheese Enchiladas (see Recipes) (2) — *bean enchilada*
Celery and carrot sticks
Brown rice (½ cup)
Fresh fruit cup
Whole milk (8 oz) — *green or herb tea*

SUNDAY
UPON ARISING
7 a.m.   2 glasses of water (preferably warm)
7:10 a.m.   Cod liver oil mixture
7:40 a.m.   Breakfast

BREAKFAST
Fresh fruit cup
Buckwheat pancakes with butter and honey — *with honey only*
Whole milk (8 oz) — *green or herbal tea*

LUNCH
Date nut bread (whole grain)
Cream cheese (1 tbsp) — *omit*
Fruit salad

Whole milk (8 oz) – *vegetable broth*

DINNER
Spinach salad
Broiled (grilled) chicken – *herring, tuna, salmon or trout*
Toasted Potato Strips (see Recipes)
String beans (½ cup)
Carrot Yoghurt Cake (see Recipes) (1 slice) – *carrot cake*
Whole milk (8 oz) – *green or herbal tea*

Dining In Restaurants – Some Cautious Reminders

We all have a favorite restaurant, a place we like to go on special occasions. 'Dining out' is a joy. So, once in a while, let someone else serve you. Let them do the dishes.

All I ask is that you use some discretion when you choose a restaurant. Does the café or dining room offer an abundance of natural foods? Inquire whether their menu includes plenty of unprocessed, unsprayed foods.

Too many restaurants and 'fast food' places rely very heavily on the use of flavor enhancers, emulsifiers, and preservative sprays.

Some restaurateurs have been spraying sodium bisulfite on fresh fruits, vegetables, shrimp, chicken, etc. The average citizen, in America, consumes 2 to 3 milligrams of sulfites each day. Where 'spraying' occurs, ingesting restaurant salads and vegetables can give a person 20 to 100 milligrams in one restaurant meal!

I maintain that the menus and dietary rules published in this chapter can do much to alleviate pain for millions of people who already have arthritis. Equally important, this nutritional program is also designed for a healthy person, as a method to help prevent arthritic ailments.

On the topic of preventing illness, I recently read a report which contained several very intelligent comments made by Dr. Williard Gaylen, President of the Hastings Institute in New York. Attributed to him were these wise statements:

'If a person followed several common sense rules for a healthy lifestyle (like proper diet, regular exercise, not smoking, routine relaxation, good hygiene, etc.) the health benefits derived would be much greater than that achieved through all the fancy medical technology of the last century.

Unfortunately, most people do not take preventive medicine seriously enough and prefer to live with their vices in the hope of being 'saved' by medical research.

It is equally unfortunate that, from the viewpoint of the medical profession, there is no profit in prevention.

Well said, Dr. Gaylen! I agree, totally. May I add that, in my opinion, the most important factor to stave off illness is a person's diet. To summarize, the best weapon can be described in just four words: Nutrition and common sense.

A Round-up Of 'Real Good' Recipes

Meals can be sheer enjoyment, and they become supreme if the person who does the cooking happens to know a few 'extra special' recipes.

Quite often, when I have eaten a very appetizing main course or dessert, I ask for the recipe. I check the ingredients – to make sure they are healthful – and then I add that recipe to my prized collection.

Recipes are to save and savor. So let me share some of my favorites with you.

By now you will know that I am not happy including meat and dairy products in dietary recommendations, so I have suggested ways to alter Dale Alexander's recipes, again in italics.

Baked Chicken Casserole – *seafood*
1 large onion, diced
1 can of tomato sauce
¼ lb of mushrooms, sliced
1 frying chicken, cut up – *substitute a mix of whitefish and salmon for chicken*

Combine the onion, mushrooms and tomato sauce. Spread one-half of the mixture on an 8 x 14-inch Pyrex baking dish. Place chicken pieces on top of this sauce. Then cover the chicken with the rest of the tomato mixture. Sprinkle with seasoning. Bake at 325°F, covered with foil, for one hour. Remove the foil. Bake again, for another half-hour. Serves 4.

Chilli Beans Supreme
1 lb pink or red beans
1 lb can of tomato sauce (passata)
½ lb ground (minced) beef – *diced carrot and red and green bell peppers*
1 large onion, diced
1 clove of garlic, chopped
1 red onion, diced, for garnish
parsley
½ tsp thyme
½ tsp oregano
1 tsp chilli powder
1 tsp sea salt

Cover the beans with water, in a 2-quart pan, and soak overnight. Next day, add the tomato sauce and simmer for one hour. Quickly fry the ground beef, without using fat, until the beef loses raw color. Keep stirring the beef constantly, then add it to the beans. In the same pan, sauté the diced onion, until lightly browned. Add the onion to the beans. Add garlic, herbs and seasoning. Next cook the entire mixture for four hours, or until the beans are tender. Stir occasionally. Add vegetables for last 15 minutes of cooking time. Serve with chopped red onions. Serves 6.

Toasted Potato Strips

These 'strips' are a treat. Instead of French fries, try this substitute. Cut a whole potato in half, length-wise. Cut each half in half again, length-wise. Do it once more, and now you'll have strips about the size of French fries. Place the pieces, skin side down, on a tray at the top of the oven. Bake (at 400°F) for about 15 minutes – or more – until they are well browned. Toast the potatoes, do not fry them. This way, there's no fat and no salt, yet the result is delicious!

Baked Fish • Red Snapper

2 carrots, sliced
2 potatoes, diced
½ lb of string beans, halved
1 zucchini squash, sliced
2 tbsp of water
1 lb of red snapper (filleted)
1 onion, diced
¼ lb of mushrooms, sliced
1 tbsp of butter – *1 tbsp of olive oil*
seasoning of your choice

Pre-cook the carrots, potatoes, string beans and zucchini in water. Add seasoning. When the vegetables are crisp and tender, arrange them in a casserole, along with the liquid from the vegetables. Sauté the onion and the mushrooms, until lightly browned. Spread them over the vegetables. Next, take thin slices of the fish and place them over the vegetables. Sprinkle seasoning on the fish. Grill until the fish turns white, which takes approximately 10 to 15 minutes. The fish tastes best when it is barely cooked. You may substitute other types of fish – like sea bass, whitefish, or flounder. Serves 4.

Mash and Smash Tuna Salad
6 hard-boiled eggs – *omit eggs and increase quality of tuna*
1 can tuna
15 sprigs of parsley, chopped
3 tbsp of mayonnaise – *soy*
½ red onion, diced
seasoning
oregano
alfalfa sprouts
1 oz Galliano liqueur (optional)

Mash and smash the eggs, with a wide fork. Mix in two of the tablespoons of mayonnaise. Add the parsley, sprinkle with seasoning. Mash and smash the entire mixture again. Add the onion, half the tuna, and more seasoning. Mash and smash. Finally, add a sprinkling of the alfalfa sprouts. Serve on slices of whole grain bread, using a teaspoonful of mayonnaise as a spread. (As an optional extra, for a little more 'smash' in the salad, you can also add one ounce of Galliano liqueur.) Serves 4.

Cheese Enchiladas – *bean enchiladas*
Sauce Ingredients:
1 can (15 oz) of tomato sauce
½ cup of water

2 tbsp chilli powder
1 tsp cumin
½ tsp turmeric
Filling ingredients:
2 medium onions, chopped
4 oz of ripe olives, chopped
2 tbsp cold pressed oil
1½ lb of Cheddar cheese – *omit*
grated cheese – *omit*
1 dozen corn tortillas – *omit*

Mix the sauce ingredients in a medium-sized frying pan. Let them simmer while you prepare the tortilla filling. To prepare the filling, sauté the chopped onions in the oil. Set the onions aside. Cut the cheese into 12 strips that will easily fit into the rolled tortillas.

Dip one tortilla into the heated sauce. Then, in the middle of the tortilla, place a heaping tablespoonful of the olive-onion mixture plus two strips of cheese (*omit cheese*).

Roll the tortilla around the filling, and place in an 8 × 10-inch baking pan. Continue this process until all the tortillas are rolled and filled. Pour the remaining sauce over the rolled tortillas. Top with grated cheese and cover with foil. Bake at 350°F, for approximately 30 minutes – or until the sauce is bubbly. The enchiladas can be assembled in the morning, and then baked just before serving. These enchiladas freeze well, for reheating later. (In all these recipes, where I refer to 'oil' as an ingredient, I mean cold pressed oil. Oils which have not been cold pressed have been heated during processing to prolong their shelf life, and some of the beneficial fatty acids have been lost.)

Toss and Fluff Spinach Salad
1 bunch of fresh spinach, chopped

6 hard-boiled eggs (mashed with a fork)
bacon bits (optional)
3 tbsp cold pressed oil
seasoning
oregano
1 tsp of cider vinegar

Pour half the oil into a mixing bowl. Use only the greenest fresh
spinach, and be sure it is dry. Sprinkle on the seasoning. Add
the eggs, plus some more seasoning. Add the diced onion. Mix
and churn. Then add the bacon bits and the rest of the oil. Toss
and fluff as you go along, sprinkling in the rest of the seasoning.
Serves 4.

Gazpacho
5 ripe tomatoes
2 tsp vinegar
1 cup of tomato juice
3 tbsp cold pressed oil
1 tsp seasoning mix
1 small onion, chopped

Blend for two minutes in a blender. Chill, in a soup tureen. If
you wish, you might also add some chopped cucumber, plus
additional onion and green pepper. You could add some
croutons, and garnish with chopped parsley. Serves 5.

Zesty Fresh Fruit Salad
½ cup of yoghurt – *add pumpkin seeds instead*
½ cup of cottage cheese
Assorted fruit
2 tbsp of honey

Your choice of fresh fruit can include peaches, pears, apricots, mango, papaya, persimmon, apples, etc. Cut the fruit into slices or chunks. Combine the yoghurt and cottage cheese and honey. Embellish your salad by pouring this mixture over the fruit.

Cottage Cheese Vegetable Soup
1 whole potato, unpeeled
1 whole yam, unpeeled
1 small onion, diced
2 scoops cottage cheese – *I would use mixed cooked beans instead and add just before serving*
1 large carrot, sliced
2 stalks of celery, sliced
1 large tomato (cut into wedges)

Cover all the ingredients, except the cottage cheese, with water. Cook slowly, in a covered pan, until tender. Remove the potato and yam. Peel and dice them, then return them to the soup. Add mixed seasoning to taste. Serve in soup bowls, over a scoop of cottage cheese. Sprinkle with chopped parsley. Serves 2.

Creative Soup
4 soup bones (avoid beef) – *omit the bones and use vegetable stock instead of water*
½ cup legumes
2 carrots
1 tomato
4 cups of water
1 onion
3 stalks of celery
parsley, for garnish

Boil the bones in water until a heavy foam forms on top. Lower the heat, and skim the soup. Add the legumes. (Or, if you wish, you can create pea soup, by adding split peas. As another variation, you can make bean soup, by using lima beans or lentils.) If you like a thicker soup, use more legumes. Next add the vegetables, and cook slowly until tender. The larger the beans, the longer they take to cook. Season to taste. Garnish with chopped parsley. You can also purée this soup. Serves 4.

Saucy Salad Dressing
2 tbsp white wine vinegar
2 tbsp honey
2 tbsp seasoning mix
1 cup of cold pressed oil

Place vinegar, honey and seasoning mix in a pint bottle. Set the bottle in a bowl of hot water, until the honey melts. Shake the bottle vigorously. Add the oil, a little at a time, shaking the bottle after each addition. Refrigerate. Just before serving, on a salad, shake the dressing again, for maximum taste appeal.

Green Garnish Salad Dressing
⅔ cup of buttermilk – *soy milk*
½ cup of cottage cheese – *omit*
¼ tsp tarragon
3 tbsp parsley, chopped
3 tbsp minced olives
½ tsp dill weed

Blend the cottage cheese and buttermilk in a blender, until smooth. Add the parsley, olives, tarragon and dill weed. Season to taste. Chill . . . and serve.

Silky's Nutty Fruit Cake

6 eggs, separated – *egg substitute*
1 tsp vanilla essence
1 tsp cinnamon
½ cup of small curd cottage cheese – *soy milk*
⅓ cup of date powder or date sugar
pinch of cloves
1 tbsp of carob powder

To use in the second step, also have ready:

½ cup of walnut chunks
½ cup of almonds, halved
½ cup of sunflower seeds
½ cup of sesame seeds
1 cup of raisins
¾ cup of dates, cut up
½ cup of figs, cut up
½ cup of prunes, cut up

First, beat the egg yolks well. Add the date sugar, a little at a time. Continue to beat. Add the vanilla, spices and cottage cheese. Beat well.

As the second step, mix the nuts, seeds and fruits into the yolk mixture. Fold in the six stiffly-beaten egg whites. Spread this entire mixture into a 7 × 16-inch Pyrex baking dish, which has been buttered. Place in a cold oven. Bake at 325°F, for 25 minutes. Test with a straw. Do not over-bake. Remove the fruit cake from the oven, and let it cool in the baking dish. This cake tastes best when it is eaten on the following day. Cut it into quarters, and store, wrapped, in your refrigerator. Store in your refrigerator. Notice that this cake contains no flour, no sugar, no salt and no fat! And it will keep fresh for weeks.

Carrot Yoghurt Cake
2 cups of whole wheat pastry flour
½ cup of wheat germ
½ cup of bran
1 tsp baking soda
2 tsp cinnamon
¼ tsp nutmeg
2 eggs beaten
1 cup of grated carrots
1 cup of yoghurt
½ cup of fresh orange juice
½ cup of molasses
½ cup of raisins
½ cup of sunflower seeds

Combine the ingredients, and beat well. Use an 8-inch square baking pan. Bake at 325 degrees F, for one hour.

Fluffy Rice Pudding
½ cup of rice (brown or white)
1 quart of milk
2 tsp of vanilla
1 tbsp of butter
2 eggs
½ cup of date sugar or raw sugar
¾ cup of raisins

Place the milk, rice, and butter in the top of a double boiler. Cook for two hours, stirring frequently. Beat the eggs well. Beat the raw sugar, or date sugar, into the eggs. Combine the hot mixture and the eggs. Slowly pour the hot mixture into serving bowls or individual dishes. Sprinkle cinnamon on top. Decorate with colorful bits or slices of fresh fruit.

The tastes and eating habits of the American people have undergone some great changes in the past 35 years. Look at the popular fads which have swept the nation: fast-food chains have promoted Mexican foods, now selling millions of tacos and enchiladas. The current rage is for croissants and quiche. Chinese restaurants have opened everywhere, tempting our palates with Cantonese, Mandarin and Szechuan cooking. And we've been invaded by the Japanese chefs, who bombard us with sushi, tempura, and raw fish delicacies.

Since we have acquired a liking for so many types of Oriental dishes, I decided to conclude this recipe section of my book by featuring:

Oriental Vegetable Delight
(a crunchy creation you can stir-fry)
½ cup diced onion
½ cup sliced mushrooms
¼ cup diced green bell pepper
¼ cup diced red pepper
½ tsp butter
½ cup Jerusalem artichoke
1 cup sliced celery
1 cup sliced zucchini squash
1 cup shredded cabbage
¼ cup mange tout
¼ tbsp natural soy sauce
½ cup whole almonds

Using a frying pan or wok, sauté the onion in butter. Add the mushrooms, and the red and green bell pepper. Sauté until lightly browned. Stir often. Add celery, zucchini, cabbage and mange tout. Keep at medium heat. Do not overcook. Lastly, add bean sprouts and Jerusalem artichoke. Season with soy sauce, to taste.

Serve with cooked brown rice. Garnish with whole raw almonds. (This recipe can be changed to substitute other vegetables which are in season.)

The beauty of this recipe – for cooking mixed vegetables, Oriental-style – is that you can do numerous variations of this dish.

Just be sure that the vegetables are under-cooked; keep them crisp. Vary the mix: try yellow zucchini, green zucchini or some of the varieties of squash now available in supermarkets and greengrocers.

For another enjoyable version, you can add sautéed scallops, shrimp, or crab.

As I was writing the above recipe, with its Oriental overtones, I was reminded of a remarkable eating experience which I had in San Francisco. Let me recall for you.

The Inspiring Story Of Dr. Dong

I was the man who came to dinner. My host was an Oriental gentleman, who had invited me to his home. He was now in the kitchen, personally preparing some Chinese food, according to an ancient recipe.

His name was Dr. Collin Dong, and he lived in a large house on Telegraph Hill, furnished with many priceless antiques. And he had a jade collection of museum quality.

Dr. Dong was then, and is now, a very respected physician. He had graduated from Stanford University, never dreaming he would become a victim of arthritis.

For seven years, after medical school, Dr. Dong practiced medicine in San Francisco. Then, at the age of 35, he was suddenly stricken with both arthritis and dermatitis. He developed excruciating pain in his shoulders and other bodily joints.

One day, Dr. Dong looked in the mirror. He had lost most of his hair. The skin on his face was cracked, swollen, inflamed. For three years he tried every conceivable method of relief. Rheumatologists he consulted placed him on aspirin, analgesics, and every form of therapy. Nothing helped.

Finally, the Chinese doctor found the answer all by himself. He tells how he remembered a certain saying found in Chinese medical literature: 'Bing chung how yup, woh chung how chut.'

Translated, that means: 'Sickness enters through the mouth, and catastrophe comes out of the mouth.'

DIET. Proper diet. Good nutrition seemed the logical way, so Dr. Dong changed his eating habits. He gave up processed foods, avoided those which had artificial flavoring, additives, preservatives.

Soon Dr. Dong returned to good health. Today he is adamant about one fact: his recovery was not a case of temporary 'spontaneous remission.' His arthritis did not occur again. It is now 48 years later. Dr. Dong is 83 years old, spry, happy, and still free of arthritic pain.

As I sat with Dr. Dong, for dinner, he told me that through the years he has treated thousands of cases of rheumatic diseases. He has told them the importance of nutrition, loud and clear.

Some years ago, Dr. Dong published his views and a collection of his recommended recipes. The volume – entitled: *The Arthritic's Cookbook.*

Research on arthritis is well underway in Japan and China. I intend to examine the progress being made by their scientists. It's encouraging that everyone now realizes that arthritis is a worldwide problem.

I hope you remember what I've told you about Dr. Dong. Because he is unique.

His is a success story which can't be denied. This man is a doctor, and a former arthritic. He knows that proper nutrition accomplished a permanent solution for his rheumatic illness.

Chapter XII
Better Health – By Process Of Elimination

Your physical fitness – your ability to enjoy life, from day to day – depends largely on whether or not your body can eliminate wastes in a normal manner.

We all suffer, occasionally, from constipation. Arthritics are particularly prone to this malady. They often report that their intestines and bowels do not function with regularity.

That's the key word: regularity. How can we achieve a 'regular' schedule and avoid constipation?

I will make some suggestions in this chapter. My research on how to combat constipation has continued for 30 years. In my first book, I devoted 20 pages to this topic, because it is such a major problem for people who have arthritis.

Noted rheumatologists conducted experiments among their arthritic patients to determine whether faulty diet is the cause of chronic constipation. Dr. Ralph Pemberton (see pages 16 and 17 of this book) restricted 'inferior-type' starches – like candy and cake from the diets of his patients. Their bowel movements improved.

Dr. A. A. Fletcher of Toronto, Canada, reported his findings in *The Journal of Laboratory and Clinical Medicine*. He recommended Vitamin B as beneficial.

According to Dr. Fletcher, constipation can be caused by vitamin deficiencies. You need Vitamin B, specifically, or else your bowel may break down and have less digestive power.

People with rheumatoid arthritis often suffer from food sensitivities which are exhibited by a variety of symptoms, including several affecting the bowel (diarrhoea, stomach cramps, bloating and constipation). An elimination diet (restricting the diet to a small range of rarely eaten foods for a period of 7-10 days then gradually introducing other foods) is the only form of diagnosis that can reveal if arthritis is related to food. Any foods that provoke a reaction can then be avoided. A restriction diet may lead to vitamin deficiency – making supplementation advisable.

Wherever I travel these days, lecturing, victims of arthritis volunteer the information that they have frequent attacks of constipation.

During a recent lecture, I told how sugar disrupts the microorganisms of the intestinal flora, which are trying to break down your food as part of the digestive process. If you block that process, you will surely experience constipation.

After that lecture came a pleasant surprise. As I prepared to leave the lecture hall, a woman walked up to me and introduced herself. She had been listening, in the audience. That day, she had traveled a considerable distance to attend the event.

'I want to thank you,' she said. 'Your previous book did a great service for my mother. Here is a letter I wrote, to express my deep appreciation.'

The letter reads:

My mother went to a medical doctor in great pain. He diagnosed osteoarthritis and X-rays showed spurs on her spine.

He gave her a prescription, but being a Carlton Frederick's fan, she was very bothered by taking drugs. So, as a last resort, she decided to go to the library, to see if she could find some helpful information, and found *Arthritis and Common Sense.*

Mom is the kind of person who has great self-discipline, and when Dale Alexander said 'no sugar' that meant no sugar – even on Christmas Day. She followed this regime faithfully until all the pain was gone, and has continued with the cod liver oil.

A few years later she went to see a nephew who is a doctor, and he took X-rays and found no spurs, and told her she had a 'photographic' spine.

Mom was born in 1899 and has a degree in Home Economics from Cornell University. Back in the 1920s, when she taught in public schools, she always put nutrition into her classes – not to the delight of her students who wanted to get on to making goodies and eating them.
Mrs. C.K.
La Mirada, California

It is moments like these – comments from grateful readers – that brighten my life, year after year. If my work is achieving results for people, then I shall continue to share my knowledge with renewed spirit.

In an effort to help constipated arthritics I have carefully designed a special formula. Printed below is a mixture of ingredients, which you can prepare in a blender, to stimulate greater regularity.

Formula To Combat Constipation
½ cup to one full cup of whole milk – *soy, almond or rice milk*
1 raw egg
2 tbsp liquid acidophilus culture
2 tbsp bran (heaping) (fibre for bulk)
1 tbsp raw wheat germ (heaping) (fibre and Vitamin B)
1 tsp brewer's yeast (level) (Vitamin B complex)

¼ ripe papaya (papain) (for digestive aid)
1 tbsp psyllium husks (fibre) (to soften stool)
1 ripe banana (whole banana, if small, or ½ large banana)
   (The above amounts, prepared in a blender, serve one person.)

My earlier remarks about the advisability of eating raw egg also apply here.

Additional Suggestions

When you feel you need it, substitute this formula drink in place of your regular breakfast. Or take it each night just before you retire. Continue drinking it, once a day, until your regularity returns.

In place of papaya plus banana, you may use six large, raw pitted prunes, or six large figs.

You may add 1 tablespoon of raw honey for sweetening.

Brewer's yeast and raw wheat germ, to newcomers, present a new taste factor. If you wish, you can begin using it in smaller quantities.

You are trying to speed up the transit time of your food as it passes through your gastro-intestinal tract. Use at least 2 tablespoons (2 x 15ml spoons) of acidophilus culture.

READ THE LABEL. Be sure to select a natural acidophilus culture. High grade acidophilus is alive with millions of hardy, viable (live) organisms.

This product should first be placed in a blender. It is not as effective if mixed in water, fruit juice or vegetable juice. And it will not be as helpful if you take the acidophilus directly from a spoon, after a meal.

Check the date on the label. The live organisms have a limited life span. After about six months 'on the shelf' the value of the product may be diminished.

The Vitamin B (in wheat germ) will gradually assist in correcting bowel-muscle tone. Bran helps to make bulky stools. Remember, you are seeking to achieve a certain type of stool, not copious amounts. For most people, one bowel movement per day is normal. However, missing a day should not cause great alarm.

> Bowel habit is a very personal matter. If you usually 'go' twice a day or once every other day and you are comfortable with that, then that is normal for you. It is a change in bowel habit that signals a problem. Dale Alexander suggests below that you establish a set time. This is an ideal and would certainly make life more convenient, but it isn't absolutely necessary as long as you have a habit that suits you.

Stool quantity may be less on a fish-type diet. Your bowel movement should be nearly odorless. Try to establish an approximate set time each day, for this natural function.

I firmly believe that both arthritis and constipation can be caused by the same dietary mistakes.

My menus, in Chapter XI, can be interchanged
You can serve the luncheon foods at dinnertime, or switch any of the dishes within the daily schedule.

The menus are designed for people of all ages. They are beneficial for young and old alike.

Some days you may be in a hurry, and you want to prepare a fast meal. Here are four suggestions, devised with speed in mind:

1. Dip some chicken or fish in egg and bran. Then, bake it.
2. Prepare a quick liquid meal, in a blender.

3. Toast a corn tortilla, topped with salsa.
4. Serve some pitta bread, heated and filled with little patties of falafel mix. (Falafel mix is now available in many grocery stores or make your own.)

I have already emphasized the value of having plenty of green vegetables in your daily diet. Let me add that I also favor sprouts. To maintain good health, we all must eat living plants. One partial answer is to start your own indoor sprout garden.

It matters not whether you use mung beans, alfalfa seeds or sunflower seeds. Sprouts are good for you. Check your supermarket, the produce section.

When preparing foods you can often use your own favorite recipes. You are not obligated to follow the recipes which I offer. You can convert your own recipes, by substituting more healthful ingredients. Here is a guide:

Your usual ingredients	*The recommended substitute*
1 cup flour	Instead, use slightly less than a cup of whole wheat or unbleached pastry flour
1 cup sugar	¾ cup of honey, plus 4 tablespoons of flour.
1 cup butter	¾ cup of unsaturated cold-pressed oil.
1 oz chocolate	3 tablespoons of carob, plus 1 tablespoon of water, plus 1 tablespoon of cold-pressed oil.
3 tablespoons of cocoa	4 tablespoons of carob, plus 1 teaspoon of cold-pressed oil, during baking.

Chapter XIII

Your Questions, My Answers

A Dialogue Between Us

By now, you have read more than 140 pages of this book. So you have probably formed your own opinion about my credibility. You may have decided that my dietary plan sounds very plausible, but you are still wondering whether or not you should try this nutritional approach.

Perhaps you have some specific questions. You are certainly entitled to seek answers about the type of arthritis that affects you most.

At the time Dale Alexander was writing his five books, the emphasis he placed on nutritional solutions for arthritis was way ahead of contemporary thinking. Since then, the science of nutrition has moved forward in leaps and bounds and on occasion caught him out. For example, his enthusiastic campaigning for cod liver oil was based on personal observation and the evidence of thousands of arthritics reported to him in letters, over the 'phone and face to face. The advice he gave was good, but his understanding of the science was at odds with the facts. It wasn't until the 1970s that the role of the omega-3 fatty acids was discovered. Even now, research is uncovering new health benefits for this nutrient-rich golden oil. Cod liver oil is undoubtedly one of the most valuable of natural remedies and an excellent example of 'grand-mother knew best'. Unbeknown to them, all the time our parents, grandparents, great grandparents and great-great grandparents were dishing out our daily dose of cod liver oil they were providing us with nutrients that help our bones and teeth grow straight and strong; promote healthy vision; protect us against heart disease; damp down inflammation and inflammatory pain; improve the condition of our skin, hair and nails; boost our immune system; promote healthy development of our unborn and newborn children; and protect against some cancers. Research is also producing evidence that omega-3 DHA may have a positive role in depression and schizophrenia.

I receive hundreds of letters. Later in this chapter, I'll let you 'read my mail' . . . and some of the matters discussed may be the very same topics that are on your mind.

I always accept any invitation from a television commentator – or from the host of a radio 'talk show' – because such interviews often give me a chance to speak directly with actual victims of arthritis. Many of the programs will announce a telephone number, so that listeners can call in. That's a great way for you to have a chat with Dale Alexander.

For instance, I recently took part in such a broadcast on Radio Station WGBS in Miami. From a tape recording which was made, some highlights are given below.

On this particular program, the host conducting the interview was Barry Young. He has a huge audience, thousands of listeners throughout southern Florida. One of the first phone calls came from a lady named Mirta. She had one main worry, and her question is one that I hear frequently.

Mirta: Does cod liver oil make you fat?

Dale: Any oil – whether it's cod liver oil, soybean oil, safflower or sunflower oil – has calories. But by taking cod liver oil my way, you are emulsifying it first. Do not, I repeat, do not take it from the spoon. (Emulsifying the oil) will take it around the liver – so that it does not act as a calorie. If it goes around the liver, it oils the skin, the joints, the hair, the eyes, makes new ear wax . . . it creates lubrication and healing power. Only if you have the correct diet which goes with the cod liver oil. It does not have anything to do with putting on weight.

> Dale Alexander's view that omega-3 polyunsaturated acids, although similar in calorie content to other fats and oils, do not put on weight is reinforced by Artemis Simopoulos in *The Aphrodite Diet*, (Vermilion, 1999). She explains her breakthrough weight-loss plan that lets you eat fat (the right kind of fat) as you lose fat.

Mirta: Another question. I have colitis. If I take cod liver oil, will that make it worse?

Dale: Once you have colitis, you must mix the cod liver oil with milk, not with orange juice. Use two tablespoonful of whole milk. Get yourself a little baby jar, put in two tablespoons of the milk, and then one tablespoon of the cod liver oil . . . and shake it into a froth. And take it thirty minutes before breakfast.

> Colitis is inflammation of the colon. As omega-3 consumption leads to the production of anti-inflammatory prostaglandins, the caller's symptoms should have improved if she followed this advice.

Barry Young: I want you to remember, everyone listening to the show today, that Dale is not going to prescribe anything for you. He's not going to play doctor with you. He's going to answer in generalities . . . He can give you some basic information about what has worked for other people. But, if you are taking medication, don't begin or end any kind of medication without talking to your medical doctor first. And I'm sure Dale will agree with that all the way.

Dale: Exactly!

The next telephone call – which I answered, on the air – was from a lady who spoke with a British accent. Her name was Valerie, and she now lives in the Miami area.

Valerie: In England, during the last war, all the adults were on rations. But the babies were given, by the Government, free rations of cod liver oil and orange juice. So, they were really ahead, weren't they?

Dale: Yes, that's very true.

Valerie: Incidentally, I drink loads of milk. I've got a gorgeous skin – not my opinion, other people's. I also have some marvelous grapefruit, which I do eat. And I'm wondering if I can substitute fresh grapefruit juice, suitably strained, with the cod liver oil?

Dale: No. You cannot mix the cod liver oil with grapefruit juice. It's ten times more caustic than orange juice.

Valerie: I was taking 50,000 milligrams of Vitamin A in capsule form. That's no good, eh?

Dale: You can use the capsules as an adjunct – as part of the energy process of your body. Capsules are surrounded by a gelatin material. It's digested and sent to the liver. It has very little to do with the oiling of your eyes or skin.

Taken on its own, I would suggest no more than 1000 mcg or μg Vitamin A per day. But as the caller was already taking cod liver oil, she shouldn't have needed an additional supplement.

This transcript of the Miami radio broadcast is just a brief sample of what was said on the air. The telephones kept ringing constantly, and I talked with listeners for two solid hours.

Your telephone calls impress me. Your inquiries are often very incisive, probing. You demand common sense answers.

Recently, my friendly mailman brought me dozens of letters. Let's 'open' a few of them and read them, together. What questions will these arthritics ask? Here's a typical letter, from a lady in Texas.

Q.   The four-hour waiting period (for drinking water after meals) is quite long. What can I drink to quench my thirst? I live in hot, humid Houston.

A.   Even during hot and sticky weather, I'm afraid my rules must still apply. But try drinking more water upon arising – ten minutes before breakfast. When thirsty, you may enjoy chewing some wet celery, or an apple.

Another suggestion is to drink a vegetable juice. Like carrot juice or freshly-squeezed orange juice – with the pulp still in the juice. Liquids like these, with low surface tension, can be assimilated more easily – without fighting the dietary oils which your food provides.

The next letter asks a question which concerns many people:

Q.   Will taking cod liver oil raise my cholesterol level any higher than it already is?

A.   Cod liver oil has no cholesterol. A normal person has a blood serum cholesterol level of 150 to 250 milligrams per

100 centimeters of blood. If you take cod liver oil properly and observe a correct diet, your cholesterol level will actually go down within a few months.

> It would be more correct to say that levels of LDL (bad) cholesterol will go down as levels of HDL (good) cholesterol rise following omega-3 consumption.

A letter-writer, who may be Italian, asked this next question . . .

Q. You never mention such foods as pasta, spaghetti, macaroni, or pizza. Can they be eaten, in moderation?

A. Of course. But it is best if they are of the whole grain variety.

Q. The only thing, Mr. Alexander, is that for years I've had this dry mouth. I can't swallow food unless I wash it down with a liquid, which is coffee, milk, or water. I drink no tea or carbonated beverages.

A. A suggestion: drink herbal tea. Perhaps one or two cups, five to ten minutes before every meal. Do this for ten days or so, and it should help.

I also recommend that you see your doctor. Have him check to determine whether you have Sjogren's syndrome. This 'dry mouth' ailment (Sjogren's syndrome) is a form of rheumatoid arthritis, occurring chiefly in post-menopausal women.

Publisher's note: The excerpts from the Miami radio broadcast quoted in this chapter accurately reflect the topics discussed. The questions and answers were edited slightly, primarily to meet the limited space requirements of this book. Minor editing also took place on the letters which readers wrote to the author, so that each question is stated concisely.

Q. What about canned soups, to which water has been added? Should they be included in the diet?

A. Yes. Soup is generally consumed when it's warm, at the beginning of the meal. Soup is considered to be a low surface-tension liquid, and that's compatible with my dietary plan.

Q. Can I have sweets twice a week?

A. Providing your arthritis is not of the rheumatoid type. It would be advisable that you try 'natural' sweets. Like sugarless, flourless cake. (See the recipe for Silky's Nutty Fruit Cake in the Recipe section.) Another route is to enjoy melon, in season.

Q. I have bursitis in both shoulders. What brought this condition on?

A. You may have imbalanced the amounts of calcium and phosphorus in your body. This could happen by eating an over-abundance of sweets. When a blood sample is taken from a healthy person, and sent to a laboratory, it will show 10 parts of calcium to 4 parts of phosphorus. Too many sweets in your diet can knock this 10-to-4 ratio out of kilter.

Another possible cause could be that you lack sufficient

> Bursitis is a painful inflammation usually caused by repeated friction and pressure on a particular joint. It can also occur in rheumatoid arthritis. It is possible that a food intolerance could be the culprit. It is also possible that the omega-3 fatty acids in cod liver oil will successfully ease the pain and quickly restore mobility to the affected joint – as indeed happened in my case.

Vitamin D oils in your bloodstream.

Q. Are the following foods allowed in your diet? Peaches?

Rice? Apricot juice?

A.   Fresh peaches are fine. Yes to rice and whole grains. Enjoy apricot juice, occasionally.

Q.   I am 78, and I'm a recent widow. I have sciatica rheumatism. Can I be helped by your program?

A.   I certainly believe that correct nutrition can have a favorable effect. Why? Because the sciatic nerve – the largest nerve in our bodies – is covered and insulated by myelin. This is a fatty substance, which can benefit from proper foods and eating habits. Also, you should be particularly careful to avoid drinking tannic-acid teas and carbonated beverages.

Q.   Is natural, freshly-made peanut butter – made on the premises, in health food stores – acceptable?

A.   Yes. Once or twice a week, that's one of my favorite snacks. Instead of bread, try spreading the peanut butter on whole grain crackers. Very tasty.

Q.   In the hospital, they keep giving me juices. Why are you against juices?

A.   I am not against reasonable quantities of vegetable juices. But I fully condemn frozen, canned, or concentrated citric juices.

Q.   I have never had any problem with my throat. But, I now talk a little hoarse. Will the oil help?

A.   For your throat condition try an emulsion of cod liver oil, rather than pure cod liver oil. Take it every night, by the tablespoonful. Do not swallow it. Let it stick to the roof of your mouth, to lubricate and heal while you sleep. Go to a throat specialist, to make sure that dryness is the only

It is important to get to the cause of any illness, however minor, or a new complaint that 'won't go away' after a reasonable period of time, so I fully concur with Dale

Alexander's advice about checking this problem out. The cod liver oil treatment may or may not work, depending on the cause of the hoarseness. I am happier with the concept of cod liver oil being swallowed as I understand its nutritional benefits.

problem. Seek medical help if you have any persistent cough.

Q.   I'm afraid to continue cod liver oil until I know if it is a saturated or unsaturated fat.
A.   Cod liver oil is a polyunsaturated marine oil. You should avoid oils that turn hard at room temperature. Such oils (found in margarine, shortening, mayonnaise) are saturated – generally with hydrogen.
Q.   How would it be if I took the cod liver oil after midnight? I always wake up during the night.
A.   That's a good plan. Simply make sure that you haven't eaten anything for approximately four hours.

Chapter XIV

Send Edible Oils To Your Joints, Not Your Liver!

As you struggle to overcome the aching pains of arthritis, there is one organ in your body which will decide your fate.

The potential 'villain' is reddish-brown in color, it weighs about 3½ pounds, and it sits astride your small intestine. The liver is sometimes called 'the pantry' of the human anatomy, because it gobbles up the choicest particles of our food, and stores them for its own use. Your liver can 'rob' your system of essential dietary oils, which are so badly needed by your arthritic joints.

The purpose of this chapter is to explain one way you can 'bypass' your liver, how you can save the edible oils and utilize them as lubrication.

Cod liver oil, when emulsified and taken on an empty stomach, can be assimilated so that 90 per cent of the oil shuttles around the liver. It does not travel to the liver via the portal vein.

In contrast, let's compare the effect of edible oils. (I refer to vegetable oils in your salad, or the fats of red meat or fish.) I maintain that with these oils, the most you can deliver to the tissues, eyes, ears and joints is only 65 per cent to 75 per cent. The liver 'steals' the rest.

Even worse, if you drink ice-cold beverages or carbonated soda pop with your meals, oil delivery will be reduced to only 5 per cent or 10 per cent.

Perhaps you have read and fully understand the facts about

digestion (page 31) and the process of 'osmosis' (page 59). Let's assume that you have also selected the right foods, from the list on pages 56–7. All these efforts on your part could be wasted, if you make mistakes in your kitchen. To prevent errors, read and remember the next few paragraphs:

> This is a fascinating theory, but not many nutritionists or gastroenterologists would be happy to publicly endorse this thinking – just yet. However, there is a sufficient ring of truth about what he says to prevent the experts dismissing it outright. I think Dale Alexander will be proved right – if only we could get these two branches of medicine working together on a research project.

Correct Cooking Techniques

How to prepare foods so you don't destroy the most valuable oils.

The first and foremost suggestion is: 'Never use a microwave oven!' The high temperatures are too hot: the oven incinerates your food, burns away the most important elements. You will destroy the very enzymes, minerals, and vitamins that your body needs most.

> The microwave oven has now infiltrated just about every home, restaurant, diner and anywhere else food is prepared in America. Familiarity breeds complacency. The fears and concerns that accompanied the advent of the microwave are now largely forgotten, but some of us are unconvinced that they are safe or such a good ideas

Frying is another detrimental method which I seldom condone. When oil is heated beyond 355 degrees, and a crusty surface forms on fried foods, then your stomach has to use more hydrochloric acid to break down the food. Your body has to supply more lipase enzyme from the pancreas to make digestion possible.

Why hasten the wear and tear on your pancreas? Eating too many fried foods makes you more vulnerable to the growth of gallstones.

Digestibility is not the only issue here. Oils heated and reheated to the high temperatures needed for deep frying and food that is cooked to crispy brownness form carcinogens. Cooking and salad oils are at their nutritional best kept in dark bottles at low temperatures and used up quickly. Cod liver oil should be taken as described in this book. Olive, walnut and other well-flavoured oils can be used in salad dressings. Evening primrose and other omega-6 fatty acids are best taken in capsule form.

Now let's consider the better ways to cook.

Broiling (grilling) is one mode of cooking that I do favor highly. It is more healthful to broil a chicken for 15 to 20 minutes rather than baking it for an hour.

Always avoid the tendency to overcook your foods. Oven baking should be done at a low temperature. Just leave the food in the oven for a longer period of time.

Whether broiling or baking, your food should be at room temperature before you start. Defrost, then wait a while before cooking.

By all means use a wok whenever you wish. The growing popularity of wok cooking is a trend that I welcome. In this method of preparing foods, you are apt to use more vegetables. That's a dietary plus, any day.

Vegetables cooked in a wok, for a short length of time do not become soggy and water-logged. Your aim should be to eat fresh vegetables while they are firm and crunchy. One advantage is that you gain more fiber content in your diet.

Steaming your vegetables is a good idea. Very few nutrients will be lost.

Better still, try waterless cooking. This will give your vegetables great flavor at mealtime. Here are a few tips on how it's done:

First, cover the bottom of a pan with diced onions. Next, add some sliced vegetables like string beans or carrots. Use medium heat, for a minute or so. Then add faster-cooking vegetables, which can include zucchini or cabbage. Turn the temperature down to low.

In this example of waterless cooking, the onions should brown lightly, adding delicious flavor to the vegetables. You'll find that the vegetables release enough moisture to steam themselves. Serve this type of food often. It's crispy, better tasting, and best for your health.

Some Fighting Words About Aluminium Cookware

Throw away those pots and pans! If they are made of aluminium, beware of those cooking utensils. They are a very real threat to your health.

Aluminium poisoning can start in your kitchen, travel throughout your body, complicate your arthritis, and then damage your brain.

Medical researchers recently performed autopsies on victims of Alzheimer's disease. They found that these patients had about four times the normal amount of aluminium in their brains.

This week, I discussed the dangers of aluminium poisoning

with an expert, Dr. H. Richard Casdorph.

Dr. Casdorph completed his extensive training in cardio-vascular diseases by serving on the staff at the Mayo Clinic. He is the author of more than 50 medical papers, and one of his recent articles is a scientific analysis on the causes of Alzheimer's disease. As a physician, he is currently associated with the Long Beach Community Hospital.

I asked Dr. Casdorph to explain his views on aluminium. He replied, most emphatically:

'I tell people that if they cook with aluminium pots and pans, it may end up in their brain.'

Dr. Casdorph offered proof of this frightening fact, by citing research work which is now being done at the University of Toronto. Doctors in Canada have discovered alarming amounts of aluminium in the brains of their senile patients.

(I'll quote Dr. Casdorph again, later in this book where I will devote considerable space to the topic of Alzheimer's.)

Every arthritic should be especially careful to avoid aluminium poisoning. Many related illnesses can be caused, unless your body maintains low levels of aluminium. For example, here is a warning which was published by the Lee Foundation of Nutritional Research in Milwaukee. They stated:

Such serious disorders as ulcers of the stomach and duodenum, cardiovascular disease, heart failure, obesity and varying degrees of paralysis of the autonomic nervous system appear to be definite consequences of aluminium poisoning.

Take preventive measures, now. I did.

I wondered and worried whether my own body was absorbing too much aluminium. So I took action to find out!

Did you know that any person can determine the exact level

of aluminium in their system by taking a very simple test? Just send a sample of your hair to a qualified laboratory. Hair analysis has become a recognized science. It is a diagnostic method which I have tried, and I recommend it as being reliable.

In my case, I sent a few strands of my hair to the Analytical Research Labs in Phoenix, Arizona. (There are many such companies, located throughout the United States. By studying the elements in your hair, they can determine the ratios of calcium, zinc, sodium, lead, iron, potassium, etc., which currently exist in your body.)

The first examination of my hair took place (in Phoenix) more than a year ago. Dr. Paul Eck, owner of the laboratory, conducted the research, and my particular interest was in the aluminium count which would register on his elaborate equipment.

Dr. Eck placed my hair sample in a test tube filled with perchloride acid. The container was then set on a carousel and spun through an atomic absorption spectrophotometer. This machine instantly measured, in milligrams per cent, the different elements found in my hair.

My reading – for aluminium – was .90 and was within the 'safe' range. Doctors have determined that there is no cause for concern until a person shows a reading of 1.5 or 2.0 in regard to aluminium.

This story about my personal experience with hair analysis has an even happier ending. I decided to pay close attention to the way my foods were being cooked. I became 'aluminium conscious' for the sake of my health.

Five months later, I sent a second sample of my hair to the same laboratory. The new reading was lower than ever. It's down to .60 and I'll make sure the reduction continues!

The Debate Rages On – Can Cookware Affect Your Food?

Many voices insist that kitchen utensils are a factor. I suggest that everyone should read a classic publication called *The Story of Aluminium Poisoning*. The authors present some excellent arguments, facts you can't ignore. For example:

They cite a test where two quarts of water were boiled in an aluminium pan. An equal amount of water was also boiled in a stainless steel pan. Then the water was cooled – and some goldfish were placed in each pan.

In six hours the goldfish in the aluminium pan were dead. The other fish were still alive.

You can conduct your own experiments. If you boil cabbage in an aluminium pot, the vessel turns black. There's a chemical reaction.

Boil cherries or grapes in an aluminium pan. If you allow them to stand in the pan for 12 hours, take a good look at what happens. Little pits or holes will be found in the pan!

A Highly-respected Dentist Joins The Fight

His words about aluminium couldn't be stronger. From his office in Maryland, Dr. Arthur F. Furman says: 'All people must make a concentrated effort to avoid additional contamination of their bodies by this ubiquitous metal.'

Dr. Furman's opinion carries real weight. He is a member of the American Dental Association, and is Chief of the Department of Dentistry at Clinton Community Hospital. His reputation is worldwide, and he has served as President of the International Academy of Medical Preventics.

I talked with Dr. Furman recently, to hear his current position on this matter. He told me: 'I urge my patients to throw away their aluminium cookware and never store food overnight in an aluminium container.'

So what shall I tell the readers of this book? What are the best alternatives? Dr. Furman and I both agreed that in your kitchen you should always use the following utensils:

Cook with:
Stainless steel
Pyrex
Enamelware
Earthenware
Cast iron
Dutch ovens

If you're a mother teaching your daughter to cook let her read this book. Then she can stay healthy. She can prevent the illnesses of middle age.

Even today, the aluminium debate wages just as fiercely. A recent statement from the Aluminium Association concentrates on the lack of hard evidence connecting aluminium with Alzheimer's disease and points to its twenty-year investment in researching possible links. It tells us that: 'To date, scientists conclude there is no evidence that exposure to aluminium or aluminium products causes Alzheimer's disease' and quotes the Alzheimer's Association statement: '. . . at this time the Alzheimer's Association does not believe that the existing evidence regarding any hypothesized relation between aluminium intake and Alzheimer's disease is sufficient to influence the use of aluminium or products containing aluminium'.

So why doesn't the issue fade away? From many years' experience of these 'scares' which so often turn out to be based in truth, I have come to understand how the system works and how vested interests put obstacles in the way of information and education. I also know that large industrial companies with big budgets can steamroller the good intentions of individuals and small altruistic organizations. It will take a lot more than these statements to persuade me to risk absorbing aluminium that I can possibly avoid.

Chapter XV

Health Problems To Watch For At The Age Of 40

Most of my readers are middle-aged. Perhaps you are enjoying those wonderful years, the mid-way mark in your lifetime.

If you feel youthful and healthy, that's all that counts. Forget about birthdays, don't add them up and become depressed.

I often smile when a person tries to hide their age. What's wrong with being 40 . . . if you're hale and hearty? I know vibrant, cheerful people who are twice that age.

Sure, on some days you may feel a bit fatigued. But you can bounce back. Live life to its fullest. You can even become a sexy senior citizen.

Bob Hope, Cary Grant, George Burns – they all found the formula for happiness in their later years. So did Lucille Ball, Helen Hayes, and other ladies.

You may be concerned about your future health. Perhaps you are experiencing some early symptoms, a few minor aches and pains which worry you. Let me devote this chapter to some optimistic news. You can prevent many illnesses, if you recognize the first warning signs, and take some simple steps to protect your stamina.

Here's the truth about your life expectancy:

Did you know that everyone could live to the age of 120?

The human body is designed to last six times the maturity of your bones. Your bones mature at age 20. (That's when you stop growing in height.) And medical science says that your bodily organs should last 120 years. Anthropologists and gerontologists (doctors who study the ageing process) all agree on this fact.

> People are living longer and staying fit and active for longer. Forty is still young. Fifty is the age when 'life begins' – as a rule, children have left home and there is a bit more money in the bank to spend on enjoying yourself and taking up new hobbies. Middle age doesn't really start until you hit 60. There's some stiff competition and some very demanding role models. Famously youthful people who belong to the 'over-50s' club include Raquel Welch, Goldie Hawn, Mick Jagger, Susan Sarandon, and Elton John. And Joan Collins, Sean Connery and Paul Newman are setting a pretty high standard for the over-60s. In one generation the concept of ageing has altered. The years ahead can truly be 'the best years of life' – but only as long as you stay healthy. There's no point living to be 100 if you are in pain, short of breath and lack strength and energy. As the saying goes: 'We've added years to life, now we want to add life to years'. Dale Alexander is right. As long as you don't smoke and take exercise, nutrition is the key to a long and healthy life.

That's an ideal attitude to keep in mind: if you are considered to be 'old' at 120, then you are still 'middle-aged' on your 60th birthday!

I told this story, half-humorously, during a radio broadcast. A lady listener didn't quite believe it. She was approaching 40, and already her health was deteriorating. I tried to encourage her, lift her spirits.

(Incidentally, the broadcast was originating from WBZ in Boston. This clear channel station, part of the ABC network, is heard throughout New England and all along the Atlantic coast. I had been invited to discuss nutrition. The talk show host was Larry Glick, who has been featured on WBZ for more than 15 years.)

One of the incoming phone calls during that program was from this worried lady. Her name was Elizabeth. She reported that she had several symptoms of 'middle age' – and I immediately questioned her about her daily diet.

Alexander: Do you wear glasses now?
Elizabeth: Yes, I do.
Alexander: What beverages have you been drinking?
Elizabeth: Well, I drink grapefruit juice, all the time.

I explained to Elizabeth that failing eyesight is often caused by consuming acidic fruit juices. Too much carbonic acid travels into the fundus vein of the eye. The costly result is a trip to an optometrist to be fitted for glasses.

Alexander: Is your hair changing color at all?
Elizabeth: My hair used to be auburn-colored. Now, it's black.

Perhaps I was able to warn Elizabeth in time. Before her hair turned gray! Acid in fruit juices and soda pop kills the tyrosinase pigment meant for your hair. (This substance is normally manufactured in the intestinal villi.)

Unless your digestive system is delivering sufficient tyrosinase to the marrow of your hair, color manufacturing stops. Simultaneously, air bubbles will develop in the marrow and your hair will turn gray or white.

Signposts of 'middle age' – like the weakening of eyesight and the advent of gray hair – are not the end of the world. Most adults can tolerate a few of these minor problems. However, when you reach your middle years, beware of more serious symptoms which could signal your need for real medical care.

If your skin becomes afflicted in any way, you should take immediate steps and seek prompt advice from a doctor. A complete physical examination, done in time, may save you from dermatitis or psoriasis.

When your skin dries out, you'll know it. First, there's the itching, then the hideous red rash. Worst of all, in psoriasis, you develop patches of scaly skin, and it can spread from your hands to your face, chest, and legs.

A typical victim was that lady, in Boston. During the broadcast, she sounded desperate:

Elizabeth: I heard you say something about cod liver oil helping psoriasis. I have a very serious case . . . and I've tried everything. I've had the ultra-violet treatment, and –

Alexander: Here's what you have to do if you want to have a beautiful skin, without the psoriasis.

It may take three to six months to get well. But you're going to have to mix the cod liver oil with milk, rather than with orange juice. Because you are sensitive to juices.

Cod liver oil will get to the skin and start healing it. It's fantastic for psoriasis, eczema, and will help stop the skin from wrinkling.

Elizabeth: Great! Okay, thank you. I'm really going to try that . . . and I'll let you know.

For years, I have recommended this same approach. It has a record of proven success against psoriasis.

> Psoriasis is an inflammatory disease of the skin that responds extremely well to dietary fish oil supplements. Cod liver oil reduces both the severity and the extent of the effects of psoriasis. The omega-3 fatty acids damp down inflammation and improve blood flow to the skin.

Vitamin A inhibits the formation of certain toxic amino acids that make the skin cells reproduce too fast. The result is less itching, reduced redness and scaling.

Publisher's note: The broadcast on radio station WBZ was recorded. Due to limited space, the quotations from that program were edited and condensed.

I shall offer indisputable evidence, throughout this chapter, that people can recover from psoriasis by correcting their eating habits. I'll relate some actual case histories, with facts on how they repaired their damaged skin.

Psoriasis deserves space in this book, because the ailment has become increasingly prevalent among arthritics everywhere. Across America, this disease torments more than 3,000,000 victims!

Unfortunately, 11 per cent of all rheumatoid arthritics also have psoriasis. So, let's discuss the problem in greater detail, and warn you about the consequences.

Psoriasis: The Ugly Prelude To Psoriatic Arthritis

By definition, psoriasis is 'a chronic, hereditary, recurrent dermatosis – marked by vivid red maculae, papules, or plaques covered with silver lamellated scales.'

Does that sound frightening? Well, the news gets worse. Very often, victims of psoriasis then develop painfully inflamed terminal interphalangeal joints. Their fingers become swollen and stiff. They have contracted psoriatic arthritis.

If you notice pain or swelling in the first joint of your finger (near the fingernail), chances are you have this very common type of arthritis. The saddest part of this story is that you could have prevented this sickness. Improper diet caused your psoriatic agony!

I can offer hope. The course of this illness can be reversed. To learn how, let's visit Texas.

There's a man in the town of Wharton, Texas, who is living proof that psoriasis can be conquered.

His story begins when he was still a teenager. He was attending Abilene Christian College, when his skin suddenly erupted with a severe case of psoriasis.

The year was 1975, and he happened to see me when I appeared on a television talk show at KPRC-TV in Houston. I mentioned how my diet was successful against skin ailments. So the student contacted me and we revised his eating habits. (Like many college students, he was consuming too many soft drinks and hamburgers. Junk food caused his system to revolt!) Psoriasis was polluting his face, scalp, chest . . . the rash was covering him everywhere except for the palms of his hands and the soles of his feet.

I heard from the young man again, four years later, in 1979. He had this to say about my advice:

Dale assured me that by following his dietary advice, I could rid myself of this disease. Within six months his predictions had come true.

Today, I still follow Dale's dietary program. I am convinced of its effectiveness. And, although I am not trained in medicine, I can see a direct correlation between what I eat and the condition of my skin.

I am greatly indebted to Dale. His untiring efforts in the field of nutrition, and his deep concern for others, were the cause of my recovery.

I have told others about this diet, with varying results. Those who have tried it have obtained the same favorable results. Others chose not to try the diet, and are in the same condition they were earlier. I urge others suffering from this affliction to try this diet.

Signed: W.W.

Wharton, Texas

Letters like that one are a joy to receive. Through the years, people from across America have written to me. In some cases, we have become life-long friends.

For example, that young Texan talks with me by telephone reporting his continued good health. (He is now married, with two children, and he teaches school near Houston.) Most important, his psoriasis has been defeated, permanently. Ten years have passed, so nobody can claim that this was temporary remission.

A National Organization Will Now Fight Psoriasis

This illness has become so widespread — with more than 3,000,000 victims in the United States. Something had to be done.

I'm glad to report that a special headquarters has been set up to help expand scientific research on this one disease. The National Psoriasis Foundation is already in action. From them, I asked for a current report on the types of therapy which are now available to the public. They'll send you a detailed description citing the advantages and disadvantages of UVB (ultra-violet light treatments), the validity of PUVA (which utilizes the psoralen drug) and other possible remedies.

I'm now a member of the National Psoriasis Foundation, and I shall support their goals. They say that psoriasis may be caused by some type of bio-chemical stimulus that triggers abnormal cell growth.

I agree with that theory. They state it, quite clearly:

A normal skin cell matures in 28 to 30 days. In psoriasis, cells move to the top of the skin in three days. The excessive skin cells that are produced 'heap up' and form the elevated, red, scaly patches that characterize psoriasis.

The white scale that covers the red patch is composed of dead cells that are continually being cast off. The redness of the patches is caused by the increased blood supply necessary to feed this area of dividing skin cells.

That description fits, very accurately, and I see that skin condition in scores of people who attend my lectures. My mail constantly includes letters on the topic of psoriasis. Right now, as I write this chapter, a man in Glendale is recovering from a bad case of psoriasis – thanks to the dietary measures he has taken.

His success story, his victory over this illness, took place very rapidly. (You might be interested to know that, as of today, it has taken me nine months to write this book. During that same period of time, this gentleman with psoriasis has had some dramatic things happen in his life.)

As an inspiration to others, here's a complete report on his case history:

I was contacted by this man just a few months ago. He is 44 years old and is District Manager of an electronics company, here in California.

Psoriasis had spread across his chest so badly that he was shedding silvery scales of skin.

By analyzing his daily diet, this man quickly realized his errors. He has been drinking a variety of acidic fruit juices, but the real culprit was ice cream. For years, he had consumed copious amounts of ice cream – a habit he now regrets.

He revised his choice of foods, and began to take cod liver oil, mixing it with milk, as the proper emulsifier.

The result? He tells it best, in his own words:

After reading your book, I am compelled to write to you.

I have not only suffered from a receding hairline but a psoriasis condition which had been diagnosed as incurable by several doctors over the past 20 years. From a medical standpoint, it was stated that the best I could hope for was to control this condition.

After following the diet outlined in your book for a period of 90 days, I have noticed my skin condition go through a remarkable change. The red sores and bleeding centers have turned to small pink ones with white centers. I know a definite cure is on it's way at last!

To read a book and have these results is close to a divine healing. I trust that others will read your book and follow your diet program and enjoy the new experience that I have with a healthy body.

Sincerely yours,

Mr. J. V.

Glendale, Ca.

When I received that letter recently, it made my day! Because it proved, once again, that a person can gain better health – without the use of drugs. Why subject yourself to oral psoralen and ultra-violet light? The best road to recovery is via nutrition.

Arthritis Is Not Caused By 'Wear And Tear' On Your Joints

Too many arthritics have been told that their aches and pains are just part of 'growing older' – as though the process of ageing is 'wearing out' their bodily joints. 'Expect some pain, and learn to live with it.'

Such a diagnosis is wrong. And don't let anyone blame your arthritis on some 'job-related' condition. Your occupation, no matter how hard you work, will not 'wear out' your joints if you are eating nutritious foods.

Whenever I meet with newspaper reporters or magazine writers, they always seem to ask about the same topic. I recall, for example, that the editors of *Healthview Newsletter* pursued this line of questioning. I quoted some of that interview in Chapter II. On this matter, they minced no words. They demanded the truth:

Healthview Newsletter: What about the wear and tear theory?

Alexander: The wear and tear theory states that osteoarthritis can be caused by overactivity in work or exercise. It's said this wears out the cushion of cartilage at the end of the bones.

This theory leaves much to be desired. For instance, for every million persons supposedly suffering from wear and tear arthritis, there are ten million people, of the same age, doing similar work, who do not have it. Why? Because they have the proper lubricating fluid in their joints.

The wear and tear theory was refuted many years ago by Dr. E.F. Rosenberg. (He reported his findings as far back as 1949, in the July issue of the *Journal of the American Medical Association.*) Dr. Rosenberg made the following points:

1. Osteoarthritis of the fingers involves only the end joints. Why isn't the whole finger affected, since all the joints are used equally?

2. Only one hip becomes afflicted. Yet, throughout the years, both hips were used equally.

3. Sedentary workers are often victims of osteoarthritis – without any signs of mechanical or physical wear on their skeletal structures.

In short, the theory just doesn't hold up.

> Exercise does not wear out the body, nor does it shorten life span, according to Dr Ralph S Paffenberger Jr. MD Professor of Epidemiology at Stanford University School of Medicines, where a group of 52,000 men who were college athletes has been studied.

Can The Climate And Bad Weather Affect Your Arthritis?

This notion is false. Weather does not cause arthritis. If geography were really the answer, why are there arthritics in sunny Florida as well as in the snow-covered mountains of Montana?

Healthview Newsletter: But don't arthritics feel worse when the weather is damp?

Alexander: That's quite true. However, is the dampness the true cause of the problem? Or is it just irritating poorly lubricated joints already weakened by friction? If weather were really the cause, then everyone would have arthritis during damp weather. But they don't.

Moreover, many arthritics who were sensitive to weather write and tell me that after cod liver oil, it no longer affects them.

For example, I got a letter from a pilot with Delta Air Lines. He had suffered from inflammation and stiffness in his wrist. Considering his occupation, it was a serious matter. In his letter, he wrote: 'After having been on the cod liver oil program for about three months, I'm hardly aware of any discomfort at all, even on cold, damp days.'

When an intelligent reader, like that airlines pilot, reports that my dietary formula has possibly solved a health problem, I feel greatly rewarded. Inspired, I work harder than ever . . . trying to spread the good news, so millions of people can benefit.

I give more lectures, more interviews. To every audience, I keep repeating the same basic message:

Proper foods and eating habits can enhance or increase the quality of synovial fluid in arthritic joints.

These are the main facts I gave, when I talked with the *Healthview* editors. I also warned them against drinking oil-free liquids with their meals.

While those editors were interrogating me, I told them to avoid drinking water, tea or coffee at mealtime. They sounded distressed:

Healthview Newsletter: What's so bad about that?

Alexander: When you eat a meal, the food is broken down into minute oily particles and mixed with the stomach juices. The heat in the stomach changes any fats in the food into tiny oily globules.

If you don't drink liquids, here's what happens . . .

The tiny oily globules (about half of them) are collected by something called the cisterna chyli. This is a passageway leading out of the stomach and emptying eventually into the bloodstream.

The oily globules travel along this passageway, get to the bloodstream and are transported to the joints. The remaining oils will travel on and eventually enter the portal vein and go to the liver.

However, if you drink an oil-free beverage with your meal, the picture changes. The beverage causes the oil globules to rupture into one large pool. Now, only about 20 per cent of them can enter the cisterna chyli, bypass the liver, and go directly to the joints. The other 80 per cent go on to the portal vein. They end up in the liver, which uses them for energy and other metabolic purposes – not as lubricants.

If you want your dietary oils to act as lubricants, you've got to get them to bypass your liver. The way to accomplish this is to avoid all mealtime beverages, except milk or soups. These two beverages cause no problems because they already contain tiny particles of oil. Hence they don't disturb the globules in the stomach.

So, to sum up, avoid oil-free beverages at mealtime. You will actually triple the amount of oils available for joint lubrication.

See my earlier comments on milk in the diet and oil absorption.

Television Remedies – Pills Being Pushed On TV

There are so many products being advertised, we are totally confused and annoyed. Arthritics are now being bombarded by TV commercials. The announcers all make the same claim: 'Relief from pain! Just try our new capsule. Our medicine is best!'

When I lecture to an audience these days, I can count on hearing questions about painkillers.

I never discuss the merits of these products, nor compare one against the other. Swallowing pills is not the way to defeat arthritis. In my opinion, they are just stop-gap measures, temporary solutions to a chronic illness.

Through the years, I have warned my readers that any drug can become addictive or dangerous. Take too many aspirin, too often, and before long you might become a victim of peptic ulcers.

It is quite obvious that I am 'anti-drugs' and there are many good reasons for my negative vote. I summarized my attitude in Chapter V of this book.

I must remind you that certain drugs may bring temporary relief for rheumatoid arthritis, yet they have no effect at all on osteoarthritic symptoms. Synthetic cortisone is one example: it is useless against knobby fingers or frozen shoulders.

May I also emphasize that I am not a solo voice when I find fault with prescription drugs. Among the leading physicians who are opposed to drug therapy is Dr. Robert Mendelsohn of Chicago, who is mentioned earlier.

At the University of Illinois, Dr. Mendelsohn served on the faculty. He has been National Medical Director for 'Project Head Start' and Chairman of the Medical Licensing Committee for the State of Illinois. Therefore, I value his opinions when he speaks out against drug therapy for arthritics.

I have discussed the drug problem with him, and we are in complete agreement. Dr. Mendelsohn and I have known each other for years. Warner Books, a division of the giant Warner Communications Company, believes in Dr. Mendelsohn. They published the soft-cover version of his famous book. It is entitled: *Confessions of a Medical Heretic.*

Let me quote just a few sentences from that book. Dr. Mendelsohn is reporting how the drug companies have spared neither time nor money in rushing their arthritis 'cures' to the marketplace. He then says . . .

Just reading the information supplied by the manufacturer of some drugs and thinking that your doctor actually is prescribing the stuff to you is enough to make you ill: 'Potent drug misuse can lead to serious results. Cases of leukemia have been reported in patients with a history of short and long term therapy. The majority of the patients were over forty.' If you read further you find that your doctor is setting you up for a possible 92 adverse reactions, including headaches, vertigo, coma, hypertension, retinal hemorrhage, and hepatitis.'

Bravo! I applaud Dr. Mendelsohn. He certainly has intestinal fortitude. He tells it like it is!

Lecithin: Should Arthritics 'Buy' This Product?

Should you purchase extracted lecithin and use it to supplement your daily diet? That's a question asked by many arthritics, because lecithin is being heavily advertised as an effective weapon to relieve rheumatic pains.

Don't buy this idea – about the healing qualities of lecithin – until you read the next few paragraphs.

I have certain reservations about lecithin, and I shall state them honestly. Research efforts are now underway, and some companies are already manufacturing 'lecithin' tablets or pills. I have my doubts whether such capsules, taken orally, can accomplish results for arthritics.

On the other hand, I do favor the daily use of 'powdered' lecithin – which is already available in health food stores.

What is lecithin? Your own body produces this substance naturally. It is a protein; some types of lecithin are found in various tissues of your body and in your blood.

Lecithin is a raw material which helps your liver to synthesize the foods you eat. In fact, some foods actually contain lecithin. Soy beans and egg yolk, for example, are sources of this protein.

For years, I have augmented my diet with small quantities of lecithin, by the teaspoonful.

For arthritics, I have already recommended that lecithin should be included in your dietary program. For instance, you will note that lecithin is one of the crucial ingredients in my Special Health Drink.

My confidence in the value of lecithin dates back many years. I learned that lecithin contains a helpful supply of B-complex vitamins, like choline.

Scientists have proved that choline can help reduce lesions. (In arthritis, when cartilages or the linings of the joints start to degenerate, lesions begin to appear.)

I studied medical papers which were published by Dr. Charles H. Best. He was the co-discoverer of insulin, in the battle against diabetes.

Dr. Best conducted many experiments, trying new diets on groups of rats. In one series of tests, he fed 20 rats a choline-deficient diet. Soon, 15 of the rats developed hemorrhagic kidney lesions and cardiac problems. He concluded that any diet for humans must contain adequate amounts of choline.

The importance of choline – and the true value of lecithin – are now being emphasized as the medical world seeks a cure for Alzheimer's disease

Lecithin is acquiring a worldwide reputation as a key factor in restoring health. For example, let me tell you about a conference which was held in Vienna, Austria. Doctors, bio-chemists, and nutrition researchers from 15 different countries were present.

The seminar continued for three days. It was the Third International Symposium on Alzheimer's disease.

I was invited to participate. I booked a flight from Los Angeles and flew to Austria, because this conference would consolidate the latest progress being made in medical research.

Arriving in Vienna, I met colleagues from Japan, Italy, the Scandinavian countries – all of us with the same goal: defeat the curse of Alzheimer's disease!

There was much discussion about dietary methods, about lecithin, and about the importance of choline. Some pharmacologists who were present now want to synthesize choline in test tubes. I hope they will decide to extract natural choline from soy beans.

Meanwhile, I shall continue to recommend that all arthritics should consider lecithin, carefully. It has beneficial qualities, but use it sparingly, with common sense.

> Lecithin is a type of lipoprotein required by every living cell and organ in the body. Although it is a lipid, lecithin is partially soluble in water and therefore acts as an emulsifying agent. It is needed for healthy fat metabolism.

Will Your Sex Life Improve After Age 40?

Your sexual activity can increase – and be far more enjoyable in the years ahead – if you just read these next few paragraphs.

I am not going to write 'advice for the lovelorn' and this book will not describe any new positions for more erotic sex. However, I do intend to reveal some facts that can increase your sexual pleasure, no matter what your age.

A healthy sex life can be yours, if you will take better care of certain glands in your body.

I'll hazard a guess that nine out of ten women have never even heard of their Bartholin glands.

Most men, by the same token, know nothing about their Tyson gland – couldn't find it if they tried.

Yet all those glands play very essential roles during sexual intercourse.

A key element for performing the sex act is lubrication. The Bartholin and Tyson glands provide lubrication – not semen – to make insertion far more pleasant. Natural lubrication is best.

You won't need gel-like products purchased in stores.

I often wondered why gynecologists do not give their patients enough information about these vital glands. Medical textbooks report that the discovery of the glands was made centuries ago.

Women can be grateful to Dr. Casper Bartholin. He did so much research, back in the year 1655, that the glands were named after him. While he was at work, in his native Denmark, another physician (across the North Sea, in England) was conducting tests among men. Dr. Edward Tyson was studying a particular gland that could secrete special lubrication during the sex act.

Let's bring this story forward – to the present day. In recent decades, millions of people did read a certain book about sex and marriage. Random House published it. The title was: *Ideal Marriage – Its Physiology and Technique.*

In that volume, if you look very closely, there is brief mention of a woman's Bartholin glands. An illustration shows that the two glands are located at the entrance to the vagina.

The Bartholin glands lie, one on each side, on the lateral walls of the vaginal introitus. Their function is described as follows:

> They manufacture a perfectly transparent, thin and very slippery mucus secretion, which, as a rule is only exuded under the influence of sexual stimuli, particularly as a result of initial psychic excitement.
>
> In normal cases, the amount of mucus is just sufficient for purposes of lubrication of the introitus vaginae, and, together with similar urethra secretions of the man, enables coitus to be carried out.

Remarkably, the same function is performed by the Tyson gland in a man. His gland is located in the corona of his penis.

A healthy male will secrete the same type of lubrication as his mate.

How To 'Awaken' Your Glands For Sexual Delight

If you and your partner want better performance, sexually, that's a happy goal. And, by now, you can probably predict the advice I shall offer.

Yes, I'm going to recommend proper diet as your best guarantee to stimulate both the Bartholin and Tyson glands. After all, we are still talking about the same subject: lubrication. The amount of natural lubrication which your body can create depends on what you eat!

'C'mon, Alexander! Next you're going to tell us that cod liver oil is good for our sex life!'

That's right! My research indicates that the Bartholin and Tyson glands require certain nutrients. They need the same fatty acids found in cod liver oil.

Every day, these particular glands must receive an adequate supply of essential fatty acids. Feed them, by eating healthful foods, as described in this book. And augment your diet with cod liver oil. Only then will you provide your body with enough linoleic, linolenic and arachidonic acid.

As Dale Alexander reports, cod liver oil can help you to a better, more active and fulfilled life! His description of the omega-3 fatty acids in cod liver oil is almost right. Linoleic acid is an omega-6 fatty acid with health values of its own. Arachidonic acid is also an omega-6 fat. Linolenic acid is the 'parent' of the omega-3 family and can convert to eicosapentaenoic and docosahexaenoic fatty acids (EPA and DHA) which ARE present in cod liver oil. EPA and DHA are more valuable to health as linolenic acid frequently fails to metabolize efficiently. I would like to add that the omega-3s in cod liver oil can also help erectile function by improving blood flow. So the omega-3s can help in two ways, both of which become more important with age as hormonal changes can affect your love life.

Don't let these glands 'dry out' – because that could lead to hospitalization and worse. There's more at stake than just sexual fun and games. If just one Bartholin gland dries up, near your vagina, it could result in cancer.

I hope that the new information in these few pages will help lubricate your sex organs. There are better things to do in bed than read a book.

For Middle-aged Readers: Some Final Advice

Facts You Need To Know About Lupus

There is one insidious ailment – with the short name of 'lupus' – which is now sneaking up on thousands of new victims every year.

At all my lectures, someone in the audience is bound to ask questions about this rheumatic illness. They want to learn more about the symptoms, and how they can cope with systemic lupus erythematosus.

Women, especially, fear this disease, because it often leaves permanent marks on their faces. Most females feel threatened. They know that lupus strikes women about eight to ten times as often as men.

The facial damage caused by lupus is a red rash, followed by marks which resemble the bite of a wolf.

'Lupus' means wolf. It's a word taken from the Latin language which aptly describes the most common symptom of this affliction. After 'wolf marks' develop on a victim's face, the rash often progresses down across the nose and into the cheek areas. By then, the markings often appear to be butterfly-shaped.

Don't get the idea that lupus merely affects a lady's vanity. This is far more than just a cosmetic problem. Lupus can be dangerous and disabling. The symptoms you may experience include muscle aches, swollen glands, nausea and vomiting.

Inflammation often occurs, which can result in kidney problems and pleurisy (an inflammation of the outer coverings of the lungs).

I maintain that lupus is a disorder of the connective tissues. It resembles rheumatoid activity of the same type that occurs in rheumatoid arthritis.

Early signs of lupus can be recognized. You may notice joint pain in your hands, wrists, elbows, knees, or ankles.

Medical science now believes that your body's immune system may hold the key as to what causes lupus. There are three main types of immune cells. All are circulating in your blood and body fluids. Their job is to attack harmful bacteria and viruses.

The subject of autoimmune disease is so vitally important, I shall discuss it in detail later on.

In the opinion of some, lupus may be related to a lack of protein or factors being present in your thymus gland. Let me report on one series of tests:

Dr. Jerry Daniels, at the University of Texas Medical Branch in Galveston, has given thymus hormone to patients with systemic lupus. He and his colleagues believe that it will correct certain immune imbalances.

(Your thymus gland, incidentally, is located in your neck close to the thyroid. Starting in childhood, this gland needs vitamins, minerals, and essential fatty acids in order to develop properly.)

Women, in their child-bearing years, are most susceptible to lupus. It has also been proven that, for some reason, lupus occurs more frequently in blacks and in certain Indian tribes than among whites.

Actually, lupus is now attacking thousands of people, worldwide. I saw the 'wolf marks' on great numbers of victims throughout Great Britain.

I hope this chapter, which was written for all middle-aged readers, has proved helpful. Next, let's turn to health problems affecting the more elderly.

Chapter XVI
Helpful Facts For Senior Citizens

When you become a bit timeworn and aged, what will be the state of your health? Most people who have arthritis also worry about other afflictions which may disable them during their senior years.

By taking a few precautions now, you can avoid many ailments as you grow older.

In this chapter, my purpose is to alert you, in advance, about certain symptoms – so you can avert a health catastrophe in the future.

It is quite possible for you to approach old age with a strong body and an alert mind. The decision is yours. When you reach the age of 65, would you rather be agile or fragile?

If you watch your diet – and eat wisely – you can prevent the onslaught of most diseases.

Even the pains of arthritis can be borne more easily than a mental illness like Alzheimer's disease. Complete loss of memory – total senility – is a tragedy we all fear.

I shall discuss Alzheimer's at some length, and warn you about the dietary mistakes which might cause your brain to degenerate. I believe that arthritics, in particular, need to know these facts . . .

Alzheimer's Disease: Brain Damage, Total Senility

The term 'Alzheimer's disease' was seldom used until ten years ago. People suffered from the illness, but it was not discussed openly.

There seemed to be a certain stigma attached to this affliction. An aged person was displaying feeble-mindedness, loss of memory, embarrassing signs of total senility.

Now, however, the public is more sympathetic, because they understand the symptoms of the Alzheimer syndrome . . . and they realize this disease can strike anyone in their later years.

Currently, this tragic form of intellectual impairment has claimed 1,500,000 victims in the United States. Alzheimer's disease is 14 times more common than multiple sclerosis.

Everyone wonders what causes Alzheimer's. In my opinion, dryness is to blame. The same lack of oils that occurs in arthritic joints is also injurious to patients with Alzheimer's. In this case, the dryness is in the sheath or coverings of the nerve tissues in the brain cortex.

The outer layer of the brain, because of dryness, develops an accumulation of abnormal fibers. Under a microscope, these changes appear as a tangle of filaments. These neurofibrillary tangles were first discovered by a German neurologist named Alois Alzheimer.

With these basic facts as background, let us now take a close look at Alzheimer's disease. A large percentage of arthritics eventually succumb to Alzheimer's, so let's talk prevention.

I believe that the dietary recommendations made in this book will also provide helpful nutrients to forestall Alzheimer's disease.

Nourish the nerve tissues in the brain cortex, with oil-bearing foods. That's one way to prevent degenerative brain damage.

You may suspect that some member of your family is slowly developing Alzheimer's. Their memory is failing, they show signs of confusion, irritability, restlessness, and agitation.

If you recognize these symptoms, have the person examined by a doctor. Unless you act, now, the victim of Alzheimer's may be headed for serious trouble.

As the illness worsens, the patient will lose judgement, concentration, orientation. Even their speech may be affected.

A physician can take an electroencephalogram. This may show a general slowing of the brain waves – and could confirm the presence of Alzheimer's.

Is Aluminium Poisoning A Factor In Alzheimer's?

Yes. There is medical proof to confirm this danger. For example, Dr. David Shore tells of tests, including autopsies: 'The brain aluminium level of Alzheimer's patients is four to six times the levels found in normal brain cells.'

Dr. Shore is a prominent researcher at Saint Elizabeth's Hospital in Washington, D.C. On the West Coast some additional warnings have been issued by Dr. H. Richard Casdorph. (See page 156.) In an interview – for *Health Freedom News* – he said:

We are literally swimming in an environment of aluminium. As you may know, aluminium ore comprises 15 per cent of the earth's crust.

Because of industrial pollution, so-called acid rain is increasing the amount of aluminium that dissolves in rain water, which becomes our drinking water.

We are being infused with aluminium. It is used commercially in baking powders, underarm deodorants and antacids.

According to Trace Minerals Systems of Alexandria, Virginia

– which is a leading laboratory in the field of hair analysis – more and more people are becoming afflicted with toxic levels of aluminium. The problem is almost endemic across America.

We are discussing an illness which is also known as 'senile dementia' . . . and senior adults have good reason to fear this affliction. Alzheimer's disease causes 60,000 to 90,000 deaths annually!

Two doctors at the Massachusetts Institute of Technology are doing some of the best research on the problem of Alzheimer's. They are a married couple – Dr. Richard Wurtman and Dr. Judith Wurtman. Quite recently, they edited a five-book publication. It is entitled *Nutrition and the Brain* – and I consider it a classic work.

Next, a news item from *The Washington Post*.

When it comes to investigative reporting, the foremost newspaper in our nation is *The Washington Post*. Read their comment, published recently: 'Aluminium, one of the most common elements on earth and long thought to be harmless, also may be implicated in several forms of human brain degeneration, particularly Alzheimer's disease.'

They based this statement on recent findings made by scientists at Cornell University, Dartmouth College, and the University of Vermont. Researchers at these institutions found aluminium in high-altitude streams – in sufficient concentrations to be toxic to fish and aquatic life, and apparently damaging to trees and plants.

The *Post* went on to say that there is 'a gathering consensus that acid rain's apparent tendency to mobilize aluminium poses a potential public health problem.'

Doctors already know that the human body stores its highest concentrations of aluminium in the lungs, liver, thyroid and brain. Antacid tablets, which we Americans consume by the millions, contain aluminium hydroxide gel. This habit could reduce your blood phosphate level.

In a person with low blood phosphate, their bones begin to dissolve, their muscles ache and are extremely weak.

Perhaps these facts have given you some helpful knowledge about Alzheimer's disease.

Low levels of the brain chemical, acetylcholine, often recorded in Alzheimer's patients, result in lethargy and poor memory, and a dry mouth. One tablespoon of lecithin granules (containing at least 30 per cent phosphatidyl chloline) may help. Elderly people are also often short of Vitamin B_{12}, so a B-complex supplement should be taken daily. Ginkgo biloba improves circulation in the brain and, as the omega-3 essential fatty acid DHA is so important to brain function, fish oil supplements may have a role. Antioxidant nutrients (Vitamins E, C and beta-carotene and the mineral selenium) will help protect the brain from further cell damage.

As well as aluminium, other substances linked to Alzheimer's include mercury (amalgam dental fillings) and the food additive monosodium glutamate (MSG). The removal of mercury fillings and avoidance of foods containing MSG are sensible moves as is the filtration of drinking water to remove pesticides which are potentially harmful to the nervous system.

Sadly, many people in their retirement years do not realise that their brain needs exercise to stay fit. Crosswords, mental arithmetic, other puzzles and quizzes will challenge the brain and stimulate the memory.

Parkinson's Disease: Trembling Limbs, and Dementia

There once was a friendly old man, an actor and comedian named Ed Wynn. He played 'The Texaco Fire Chief' in the early days of television.

In his later years, whenever Ed Wynn appeared on TV, we

watched with compassion, because his hands were trembling, he walked hesitantly, and he spoke with great difficulty. Ed Wynn was a victim of Parkinson's disease.

The staggering truth is that 1,000,000 people throughout the United States now have this vicious affliction. Every year, more than 50,000 Americans learn they have Parkinson's!

This disease affects both men and women, mostly those who are 40 years of age or older.

Dr. James Parkinson, a London physician, first described this illness. His research was done in the year 1817, and the problem has been growing ever since. Now, in the next few pages, I'll try to give you a current picture on where we stand.

First, you will need to know something about your basal ganglion. In anatomy, the ganglion is a group of nerve cell bodies, and we are interested in those which are located next to your brain stem.

Basically, Parkinson's is a brain disease. Some doctors compare it to 'hardening of the brain arteries', and a concentrated effort is now underway to find a cure. The National Parkinson Foundation has been established, based in Miami, Florida.

To protect yourself, and your loved ones, you should learn the early symptoms of Parkinson's. There is more involved than just noticing tremors and slowness of movement.

Other manifestations of Parkinson's are easy to identify. Researchers, at the Foundation, have published this list:

1.   Victims of Parkinson's have episodes of 'freezing', where they have sudden difficulty in walking. They freeze, particularly in moving through a doorway or in turning.

2.   They experience dementia, and show a decreased memory for recent events.

3.   They exhibit periods of depression.

4.   Some patients sweat excessively, and have oily skin. May have visual problems simultaneously.

5.   Cramps may occur. Plus a burning sensation in the thighs or legs.

6.   Another indication is when the person has low backache, accompanied by poor posture.

If you encounter any of the six symptoms listed above, you should seek a doctor's advice immediately.

The final problem we ought to discuss is speech impairment caused by Parkinson's. This illness often affects the muscles necessary for speech production.

Muscles in the mouth, cheeks, jaw and lips fail to function properly. Rigidity of the facial muscles makes even smiling difficult. The patient may have reduced breath support. This is caused by rigidity of the chest muscles. Therefore, the person will have low volume and a weak sounding voice.

Proper Diet Can Help – Defeat Dryness As First Step

I believe that the same dryness experienced by arthritics is also dangerous to anyone with Parkinson's.

Dryness – in the basal ganglion, next to the brain stem – should be avoided at all costs. Food nutrients are needed to help your brain make acetylcholine. Your diet should supply choline. As one rich source, you should eat more fish.

Lecithin also contains choline (as phosphatidylcholine). So, act accordingly.

Some doctors report that Parkinson's is caused by an oxidative process. To gain a degree of protection, you could try antioxidants such as Vitamins C, E, B1, B5, and B6.

The antioxidant vitamins are A (beta-carotene), C and E. The mineral selenium also has antioxidant properties and I would add this to the list. The B-vitamins are active in nerve health and I would recommend them for this reason.

If you can detect this disease early – and seek medical help – the patient can survive for many years.

In addition to trembling fingers and tremors, watch for these signs: the victim develops a stooped position and a slow, shuffling gait. He or she may acquire a diminished facial expression, and may hold arms fixed at the side when walking.

To conclude our discussion about Parkinson's disease, let me simplify the main facts . . .

1.   Your brain works because your nerves talk to each other, with chemicals called neuro-transmitters.

2.   Neuro-transmitters are manufactured in your body from nutrients in the food you eat.

As scientific research continues, it may well develop that good nutrition is the ultimate answer to Parkinson's.

Why have I devoted so much space in this book to the subject of Parkinson's? Because nearly 5 per cent of all arthritics eventually develop this illness. Let's start working, now, to reduce that figure!

At almost all my lectures, several people in the audience asked questions about Parkinson's disease.

'Is it inherited?' No. There is no medical evidence to indicate that this illness can be passed from generation to generation. Also, the ailment is not considered to be contagious.

'Is exercise advised?' Yes, some doctors do recommend a program of special exercises, to reduce rigidity of muscles, and to prevent atrophy.

'Is any medication available?' That question opens a whole controversy. As you know, I am quite adamant against the use of drugs. However, some physicians believe that patients with Parkinson's are suffering from a lack of dopamine. To replace this chemical – to stimulate the nerve cells in the brain – the current prescription is usually for L-dopa.

I'll leave the choice up to you. Improve your diet for permanent relief. Or it's L-dopa.

There is no hard evidence to show that nutritional measures can treat Parkinson's, but everything that has been learned about nutrition in the past 50 years tells us that the diet must have a role in its prevention. Optimum nutrition is our best protection against any degenerative disease (Parkinson's is attributed to degeneration). The body can function better and last longer if it is supplied with all the nutrients it needs, in the same way that any machine can be kept in good working order if it is well maintained. Every single survey in the past decade has shown that even people who think they eat a balanced diet are unlikely to meet all recommended daily intakes of vitamins and minerals. As with all drugs, L-dopa has side effects, notably nausea and sometimes involuntary movement and mental disturbance.

At Columbia University Department of Neurology, physicians gave high doses of Vitamin E (1800–3000 IUS) and Vitamin C (3000–6000µgs) daily to Parkinson patients and followed for ten years. Those consuming antioxidants did not require drug therapy with L-dopa as early in the illness as those who received no antioxidants.

Cancer Arthritis: Inflammation, Followed By Tumors

Anyone, after taking a physical examination, is nervous. If the doctor even mentions the word cancer, the patient becomes terrified.

So, very few people have been told that they have 'cancer arthritis' – the term is seldom used. But the disease exists.

I intend to describe the symptoms, and reveal the history of this illness. Knowledge can keep you forewarned.

Cancer arthritis was really discovered – and was clinically studied – more than 25 years ago. The two doctors who deserve credit for its research were associated with a hospital in Copenhagen, Denmark. Dr. Brynjolf Strandberg and Dr. Neils Jarlov reported their findings at the Third International Congress of Physical Medicine, held in Washington, D.C., in 1960.

They conducted their tests among 53 patients, all of whom were hospitalized. The patients had been diagnosed previously as suffering from rheumatoid arthritis.

Dr. Strandberg determined that rheumatoid arthritics often have inflamed joints, and lesions which later developed into tumors.

In these patients, the protein levels of their blood was in disarray. Their alkaline phosphatase level was elevated. Their albumin-globulin ratio was reversed. Normally, they should have had two parts of albumin to one part of globulin. Instead, these 'cancer arthritis' patients had the opposite reading.

Stated in more simple language, the early signs of this illness manifest themselves as follows: you might notice swelling, stiffness and restricted movement, first in the small joints of the fingers, then in the toes, foot, elbow, knee, shoulder and hip.

Other symptoms include inflammation and fatigue. As lesions grow worse, they progress toward becoming tumors. Dr. Strandberg concluded: 'Rheumatoid arthritis may be the first clinical sign of cancer.'

When I learned that cancer and arthritis might be closely related, I began attending conferences to study this combined threat to everyone's health. A dozen years ago, I joined the I.A.C.V.F. – the International Association of Cancer Victims and Friends.

(Later, I was elected Vice President of that organization, and served for three years. I am also a member of the Cancer Control Society. They have 30 chapters, nationwide. This year, I lectured at their 12th annual conference.)

A Movie Star Dies From Cancer Arthritis

This illness is not something new. For example, it claimed the life of a famous personality, Rosalind Russell, who died in 1976. If you remember some of the newspaper articles, they reported that her death was due to cancer rheumatoid arthritis.

While I was writing this book, I contacted the National Cancer Institute. I was seeking their latest recommendations on how to prevent cancer. And here's a very interesting development. They are suggesting that proper foods can protect your health!

'Current evidence suggests that by choosing carefully and eating a well-balanced diet, you may reduce your cancer risk.'

They said it, not I. But, naturally, I am in total agreement with their nutritional approach. Let me quote exactly what they recommend:

Eat a variety of foods every day. Include fresh fruits and vegetables, especially those high in Vitamin A and C . . . such as oranges, grapefruit, nectarines, cantaloupe, and honeydew melons.

(I can only add that you should eat these foods, and chew them well.)

They go on to say:

Choose leafy green and yellow-orange vegetables. Like spinach, kale, sweet potatoes, and carrots, as well as cabbage, cauliflower, broccoli and Brussel sprouts.

Eat foods with fiber, such as whole grain breads and cereals; a variety of raw fruits and vegetables, especially if eaten with the skin; beans, peas, and seeds.

Does all this sound vaguely familiar? Of course it does. You've been reading the same advice since page 1 of this book.

To prevent cancer – and cancer arthritis – you can also rely on certain vitamins. The United States Department of Health and Human Services has voiced their favorable opinion about essential vitamins.

In a booklet prepared in cooperation with the National Institute of Health, they emphasize the role that vitamins should play in your daily diet.

Quoting them, I also agree with these facts:

Scientists have found some relationship between a lack of certain vitamins – A and C – and cancer. For example, diets low in Vitamin A have been linked to cancers of the prostate gland, cervix, skin, bladder, and colon.

You can get all the vitamins A and C your body can use if you choose two helpings daily from the same fruits and vegetables that are in a balanced diet – dark green vegetables, yellow-orange vegetables, and yellow-orange fruits.

If you are worried about contracting cancer, these past few pages have given you a clear guide on how to minimize your risk.

> Vitamins A (in its vegetable form, beta carotene) and C are two of the antioxidants mentioned in the section on Parkinson's Disease. To these can be added two more: Vitamin E and the mineral selenium. The antioxidant nutrients are major weapons against disease and ageing. Called free radical scavengers, they mop up harmful

chemicals that damage cells by oxidation. Research has confirmed that they do have a positive role in the fight against cancer and has led to the recommendation that everyone should eat at least five portions of fruit and vegetable every day. As most people's diets fall far short of this, it is an argument for supplementation. Certainly supplementation with Vitamin E, which is also heart protective.

Dale Alexander would have been delighted, although probably not surprised, to find that fish oils are now also believed to protect against cancer. Statistical data shows that about 60 per cent of women's cancers and 40 per cent of men's cancers are related to nutritional factors and studies to date suggest that fish oil can be used for both prevention and treatment of cancer. Although there is no clear mechanism to explain their anti-cancer effects, knowledge of fish oils' role in cell function suggest several possibilities:

* Alteration of cell membrane composition to affect the cells' response to growth factor, hormones and antibodies
* Inhibition of the prostaglandins that can stimulate the growth of tumors
* Strengthening the immune system
* Interference with hormonal profile (as in breast cancer)
* Tumor cell toxicity – probably by causing lipid peroxidation in tumor cells

Now let's turn to another health problem, one that haunts millions of people during their senior years.

High Blood Pressure: The Invisible Disease

You don't even know you have it. This illness gives you no outward signs – no swollen fingers, no painful symptoms to warn you of trouble. High blood pressure can creep up on a person, unnoticed.

Only one-third of the people who have this ailment are being treated. And half of those patients don't follow their physician's advice rigorously enough to bring their blood pressure under control.

Because it is essentially painless – until you are felled by a stroke or a heart attack – you tend to ignore your blood pressure. That's a bad gamble!

Sixty million Americans are seven times more likely to have a stroke than their fellow citizens, just because their blood pressure is higher.

Most doctors agree that high blood pressure is usually caused by one of the three s's: salt, stress, or smoking.

One out of four Americans could really benefit from therapy – their blood pressure has elevated to an unacceptable level.

I shall have much to say, shortly, about sodium in your diet. Basically, the key rule is: 'Don't use that salt shaker!'

Most adults, especially elders, now eat about 10 to 12 grams of sodium chloride each day. The sad fact is, your kidneys were created to deal with only one tenth of that amount.

In order for your body to excrete the salt you will need more water in your system. The salt must be diluted. By the time you become a senior citizen, your body is automatically retaining 5 or 10 pounds of extra water to aid in the dilution of salt.

Pressure must be exerted, by your own vascular system, to force out the sodium excretion. This may place a burden on your kidneys. The added work causes your blood pressure to soar.

Stress: Doctors Now Call It 'Hypertension'

If the patient seems nervous and distraught – causing a rise in blood pressure – it is now popular to blame it all on hypertension.

'Here's a pill to calm you down.' Why? Why do we always turn to drugs?

My objection to oral medication is not just a solo crusade. On this matter, my views run parallel with those of Dr. Cleaves Bennett. He is one of the nation's foremost experts on hypertension.

Dr. Bennett began his career in New York State, by graduating from the University of Rochester School of Medicine and Dentistry. After earning his M.D., he became a nephrologist – a physician specializing in kidney diseases.

Most recently, Dr. Bennett wrote an important book. It was published by Doubleday and Company (New York). Speaking forcefully, the title is: *Control Your High Blood Pressure Without Drugs!*

This learned doctor says it quite plainly, in one sentence: 'High blood pressure can and should be controlled by good nutrition, exercise, and stress reduction.'

Dr. Bennett describes high blood pressure as 'the silent killer'. So heed that warning, now. Damage can be going on inside you, where you can't feel it. Inside your arteries, inside your kidneys, even inside your eyes.

He concludes: 'That shortness of breath that stops you when you walk, or wakes you at night, is another sign of blood pressure out of control.'

He outlines a twelve-week program that attacks the causes of hypertension on three major fronts. The three key answers are: diet modification, stress reduction, and simple but regular exercise.

For added evidence, let's meet another doctor:

Dr. Robert Downs practices in Albuquerque, New Mexico.

He, too, has done extensive research on many circulatory diseases, including high blood pressure. I have known Dr. Downs for nearly ten years, and have met with him for conferences about nutrition. As an author, he writes a popular column on health topics.

Dr. Downs received nationwide attention not long ago when he discussed garlic as having possible therapeutic value. He was interviewed by a writer from *Bestways* magazine, which published these facts:

Bestways: What do you use in treating high blood pressure patients?

Dr. Downs: Garlic works to reduce hypertension. Because of the oil components and chemicals which stimulate a certain prostaglandin in the body to shift the sodium balance out of the cells.

It (garlic) acts as a cellular diuretic and reduces high blood pressure in a mild way. Because of the oil components in the garlic, it inhibits the platelets from aggregating, thins the blood, provides less risk of blood clots and a better blood flow.

I respect Dr. Downs, and I concur with his findings which favor garlic.

Notice that he mentions a prostaglandin. It is a term which is of fundamental importance to all victims of arthritis. You will learn more about prostaglandins in the next chapter – how they may control inflammation and reduce arthritic pain.

Prostaglandins are of such significance to you, let's take a moment to explain what they are. This is the definition, from *Dorland's Medical Dictionary*:

PROSTAGLANDIN – Any of a group of naturally occurring, chemically related hydroxyl fatty acids that stimulate contractility of the uterine and other smooth muscle and have the ability to lower blood pressure, regulate acid secretion of the stomach, regulate body temperature and platelet aggregation, and to control inflammation and vascular permeability; they also affect the action of certain hormones.

Medical research on prostaglandins is now a major activity in laboratories throughout the world. (See Chapter XX.)

But, right now, let's return to the subject of plain, ordinary garlic. Is it conceivable that the tiny cloves from this strong-smelling plant can actually reduce high blood pressure?

Yes, I agree with Dr. Downs. Garlic can help. Extractions (taken from raw garlic) are available in three forms: capsules, tablets, and liquid garlic.

I believe that the capsules are best. Take them with your food, but, remember, don't wash them down with water.

You may find, however, that you need as many as six capsules per day in order to make some headway in reducing your high blood pressure.

Perhaps a better idea is to eat more raw garlic. Grind it up into your salads, just one or two cloves of garlic a day. Rub your salad bowl with them. Add garlic to spice up some of your recipes.

Arthritics Have Blood Sludging, Poor Circulation

'Blood sludging' is a rather vague description that has more recently been described as 'blood stickiness' or more properly as 'platelet aggregation'. Blood platelets (officially known as thrombocytes) are manufactured in the bone marrow and discharged into the blood, where they are responsible for blood clotting. Without them, we would literally bleed to death following injury.

Blood clots in already damaged or narrowed arteries, however, can block blood flow and therefore starve the heart of vital oxygen leading to a heart attack. Treatment of patients at risk of heart attack targets reduction of platelet aggregation with aspirin or omega-3 fatty acids, EPA in particular. There is a weight of evidence to demonstrate that fish oils reduce any tendency of the platelets to stick together and also help dilate blood vessels. Fish oils are not linked with gastric problems associated with aspirin.

Magnesium is a mineral whose intake is often inadequate. In many people at risk of heart attack, the amount of magnesium in the body tissues is not only depressed but actually deficient. When the heart muscle is deficient in magnesium it is unable to retain potassium, so also suffers from potassium deficiency. Magnesium supplementation is associated with several heart health benefits, including protection against atherosclerosis (thickening and hardening of the arteries), irregular heartbeat and angina.

Most patients with arthritis also find that their circulatory system is not functioning properly. Blood sludge is evident – and that can cause your blood pressure to rise.

To prevent blood sludging, I recommend a diet which is high in magnesium content. This will help to dilate your blood vessels.

Among the best foods containing magnesium are legumes, nuts, and whole grains. You can also gain magnesium by eating fish and lean meat. In these last few pages, I have given you the current thinking about high blood pressure and related ailments. To summarize: SALT is your worst enemy.

To avoid salt, don't eat cold cuts, and don't use salty

condiments, like catsup (ketchup). If you are fighting high blood pressure, do drink more water. Have a glass of water ten minutes before a meal, or drink it at least three to four hours after a meal.

Water will hydrate your system. It will help your body eliminate excess salt, via your kidneys.

This entire chapter has been directed toward senior citizens, older people who are ailing. I could cover many topics. When you age, you become prone to a wide variety of health problems: failing eyesight, loss of hearing, insomnia, constipation, etc.

But there is one serious illness which I feel compelled to discuss. Many arthritics simultaneously suffer from diabetes. For several pages, the villain has been salt. Now, let's consider the dangers when you eat too much sugar.

Diabetes: Too Much Sugar Leads To Insulin Shots

I have real sympathy for any person who faces needle injections, day after day. Diabetics, taking insulin, are forced to endure this treatment – or risk terrible consequences.

In the United States today, diabetes is the third largest cause of death. The other two killers are cardiovascular disease and cancer.

Grim statistics also prove that vast numbers of Americans are now losing their fight against diabetes. Because of this illness, they require surgery. It's a shocking fact that each year there are 60,000 leg amputations performed.

This gruesome toll of limbs is just one tragic result of diabetes. Across America, this same disease is the leading cause of blindness.

We know why people develop diabetes. The sugar chemistry of their body has been upset. The amount of glucose in their blood will vary, depending on what the patient eats, and their blood sugar level will rise abnormally.

Diabetes is one ailment which is diet-related, and most medical doctors immediately warn their patients to change their eating habits. 'Reduce your intake of sugars, that's imperative!'

I have always limited the amount of sugar that is allowed in my dietary program. All the menus and recipes which I recommend for arthritics are low in sugar content. Therefore, my nutritional ideas can also be very beneficial for anyone who has diabetes.

Repeatedly, throughout this book, I have warned against eating too many sweets. Instead of sugar, I have suggested that you should use natural substitutes in most of the recipes.

The foods I have listed – and the proposals I have made as to when you should drink beverages – were carefully designed so that you would place the least possible strain on your pancreas. That's the goal, for arthritics and diabetics. Protect your pancreas!

The medical profession agrees that diabetes is a malfunctioning of the pancreas. The organ is not able to cope with the amount of sugar which the digestive system is delivering to the pancreas. Therefore a diabetic's blood soon develops too high a level of glucose.

You will notice that my 'Special Health Drink' (on page 116) includes brewer's yeast. This product has often been called 'the poor man's insulin' – it is so healthful for diabetics.

Specifically, brewer's yeast contains a generous supply of B-complex vitamins. They can help correct the overabundance of sugar in a diabetic's bloodstream.

Many arthritics – as they grow older and reach their senior years – must also fight off the scourge of diabetes. I often hear from people who have both maladies, simultaneously.

By complete coincidence, while I was writing this chapter, my mailman delivered a packet of letters. My publisher in

Connecticut forwards any mail which is addressed to me, and look what came in this week . . .

This is the actual correspondence; it is from a nice lady who was the victim of two illnesses. She wrote:

Dear Sir:
I am sending this letter to you (the Publisher).

I want Dale Alexander to know what his program on nutrition for arthritis and diabetes has done for me. I suffered severely for a year with arthritis of the spine, in my neck and up the back of my head. It was so severe I could not function well enough to accomplish anything.

By an act of God, I was presented with a book called *Good Health and common Sense* written by Dale Alexander. I followed the chapter on arthritis, taking cod liver oil, brewer's yeast, etc.

Within a few weeks I was much better, and now after five months I am free of any arthritis. It works. All the drugs I took prescribed by doctors did no good.

Also, I've been a diabetic for 30 years, and I've had to use insulin. The brewer's yeast has definitely lowered my blood sugar. I've cut my insulin 10 units.

Mr. Alexander is a king in my book. I thank you, Dale Alexander.

Sixty-one years old and feeling great . . .
Signed
M.L.
Viola, Illinois

I truly appreciate those warm words of praise. They reinforce my theories about nutrition. I receive countless letters, unsolicited testimonials.

But I am also a realist. No matter how many letters are sent to me, the medical profession will still argue that my dietary program is not valid. Doctors will say that my research work has not had any clinical tests. Ladies and gentlemen, just read the next page . . .

Chapter XVII

Believability: Are My Theories Tested Or Contested?

The title of this chapter asks a blunt question. And I intend to answer it – publicly, and in print.

I know, full well, that my dietary program has been soundly criticized. Charges have been made that my nutritional procedure has not been adequately tested. According to some members of the medical profession, my dietary plan is an unproven theory.

On more than a few occasions, my credibility has been challenged. In the past, I have taken this verbal abuse very quietly. But now, in this chapter, I shall reply!

When my first book gained wide acceptance by the public, a storm of controversy developed. It was led by some rheumatologists in Massachusetts. They spoke out, from the Boston area. They spread their opinions in an attempt to counteract mine.

The issue was whether or not there was any oil in the synovial fluid of human beings. The Boston doctors claimed such oil, in the joint cavities, did not even exist.

Unable to gather sufficient amounts of synovial fluid from humans, these arthritis 'experts' were conducting their tests with synovial fluid taken from cows.

Based on bovine fluid, they were making flat statements concerning human arthritics.

On this matter – the type of testing – I'll let you decide about their credibility.

Perhaps they should not be harshly blamed. At that time, in the late 1950s, certain scientific equipment had not yet been invented to identify the oils.

I was convinced, of course, that these oils were a reality, and their effectiveness could be increased through proper diet. My first book also explained how and why cod liver oil was an essential weapon.

My critics prevailed, however. They frightened many doctors, caused them to reject the book.

Seeking support, I approached the American cod liver oil industry, urging them to test my theories in their laboratories. Supposedly, they knew their product and could scientifically prove its benefits for arthritics.

I was discouraged. My efforts to arrange a fullscale clinical evaluation had apparently failed.

But now comes the good news . . .

The facts I am about to reveal have never been told before. I saved this outstanding development – so I could publish the facts in this book.

My dietary program has been tested, on human patients, with excellent results.

The clinical evaluation was conducted secretly – without my knowledge, and without any persuasion on my part.

It happened because thousands of arthritics, in England, were reading my first book. Favorable articles began to appear in newspapers. Letters from grateful arthritics impressed some key scientists in London.

A study was commissioned, and the research work was done at the Charterhouse Rheumatism Clinic. A group of 103 patients agreed to participate, and the tests would continue for 20 weeks.

Dr. Harry Coke was the scientist in charge of all these experiments. With each patient, he began by aspirating fluid from their afflicted joints. With a needle, he withdrew synovial fluid from their knee joints.

The aspirated samples were sent to a laboratory in Hull, England. There, gas chromatography was used to analyze the lipids – the oils.

The chromatography equipment had been invented recently. (In fairness, I add that this scientific device was not available when the Boston doctors did their earlier research.)

All the patients in London had oil in their synovial fluid, from the very start.

As part of this clinical evaluation, the 103 patients were all given cod liver oil: one tablespoon per day, for 20 weeks.

Then each patient was aspirated again. Gas liquid chromatography again measured each sample – drawn directly from the arthritic joints. The results were outstandingly good. In only 20 weeks, the oils had increased from an average of 0.12 per cent to 2.58 per cent. In effect, the patients had increased more than twenty-fold their supply of beneficial oils!

I am humbly indebted to Dr. Coke and his staff, for their diligent work. The evidence is now on the record. I rest my case.

That medical evaluation, at the Charterhouse Rheumatism Clinic, was later reviewed by other doctors and arthritis authorities.

One such expert is Dr. Verna Wright, renowned as a Professor of Rheumatology at the University of Leeds. Dr. Wright was asked to comment on what Dr. Coke had proved by these tests.

Here is just one statement made by Dr. Wright: 'The most exciting concept is that cod liver oil may be a precursor to prostaglandins.'

What a happy prospect that is! Other researchers around the globe should respond to that cue. The medical world is currently investigating fatty acids (prostaglandins), and cod liver oil should be included in their future tests.

With my views substantiated, I shall continue my research work, more actively than ever.

The accomplishments at Charterhouse Clinic have sustained me, and I am most thankful for the confidence that they showed in my nutritional theory.

I have struggled for 30 years, trying to secure some kind of support from rheumatologists here in America. My countrymen, I'm sorry to say, are still skeptical. I refer to those doctors in 'organized' medicine, those who keep insisting that my dietary program is a myth, unable to help arthritics.

Until quite recently, they claimed that fish oil as a therapeutic substance was a fish story.

But now, this year, there are encouraging signs that negative attitudes are changing. Very important experiments have begun – in Boston, U.S.A.!

Heartening news! It seems that arthritis sufferers in Britain have made up their own minds and have voted to take cod liver oil. In a bizarre set of circumstances, the Department of Complementary Medicine at the University of Exeter conducted a survey into complementary therapies for the treatment of arthritis. It seems that a popular women's magazine erroneously reported that the University was recruiting patients for just such a trial. The response was so high (almost 3,500 applicants) that it was decided to seize the opportunity. From responses to a purpose-designed questionnaire, cod liver and fish oils were the only remedy perceived as effective. The report supported this finding by quoting that 'at least six controlled trials support the notion that fish oil is effective'. This is a victory for common sense.

At Last! Research Being Done To Test Fish Oils

Finally, after all these years, rheumatologists and respected doctors are starting to acknowledge that oil-bearing diets might affect arthritis.

I have been heartened and inspired anew, thanks to something that happened at a meeting of the American Rheumatism Association.

The foremost arthritis experts from throughout the United States gathered in Minneapolis – in June of 1984 – to discuss the latest advances being made to treat this disease.

Nearly 500 medical papers and reports were presented at that conference. New scientific projects were revealed. One analytical study they announced is truly significant. Doctors doing research work in Massachusetts described their successful tests.

I immediately telephoned the Veterans Hospital in Bedford (near Boston) to seek full information. I spoke with Dr. Edgar Cathcart, who is in charge of the experiments. He is Director of the Geriatric Research Educational Clinical Center.

Dr. Cathcart and his colleagues, after months of work, accomplished a successful series of laboratory experiments. They set out to determine the value of fish oil versus corn oil in regard to inflammatory diseases such as collagen induced arthritis.

The expert staff included biochemists, a veterinarian, researchers, lab technicians – a highly trained team. They used as many as 160 mice during these dietary experiments.

I asked Dr. Cathcart to describe the exact way in which these tests were conducted. 'What did you do, as the first step?'

He told me:

We began by injecting a collagen material into the ears of the mice. We created an arthritis-like condition in the animals.

The mice were then divided into two groups. One group was maintained on a diet which contained 7 per cent corn oil. The other mice were fed the same diet, but instead of corn oil, we augmented their food with 7 per cent of fish oil.

(The fish oil selected from these experiments was taken from a species known as Menhaden. This is a shad-like fish, caught off the Northeastern coast of New England. I just wish they had used codfish. I am a bit prejudiced toward cod, as you know.)

Dr. Cathcart continued his description of the experiments, as follows:

After 23 days, we tested the blood of all the mice. Those mice who had been given fish oil experienced better immunity protection.

Here was proof that dietary fat can modify the outcome of autoimmune diseases!

In the paragraphs above, I have purposely given a simplified description of these experiments. I've tried to use non-technical language. Actually, these tests were very elaborate and scientific. From the mice, macrophages were harvested. Adherent cells were cultured for 24 hours. The prostaglandins and the thromboxanes were measured by radio immunoassay. So this evidence is accurate, beyond question.

Yes, the medical profession is ready to agree that fish oils can favorably affect arthritis. The importance of marine oils is now being confirmed. The rheumatologists have authenticated these facts in their own scientific laboratories.

It's true that the experiments in Boston were performed with mice, not humans. But the day is soon coming when dietary tests will be extended to hospital patients. Human volunteers are certainly available – like those arthritics who took part when my diet was studied at the Charterhouse Clinic.

Throughout the United States, people are now eating more fish than ever before. This, too, is a very good omen for the health of our nation.

I have always recommended fish as a food. Now, several prominent writers have proclaimed the many advantages, urging you to add fatty fish and shellfish to your own diet.

Recently, *The New York Times* published a major article listing the benefits of eating more fish every week.

Human Beings Require The Fatty Acids Found In Fish

Cardiologists are now suggesting that we should eat fatty fish and shellfish at least three times a week. This would have a protective effect on our hearts and blood vessels.

I agree. Occasional meals featuring fish can help lower your cholesterol level. Therefore, you will have less risk of blood clots. Minimize your chances of having a stroke.

The special report in *The New York Times* – in their column on Personal Health – was primarily written for readers who had cardiovascular problems.

May I remind you, however, that arthritics are closely involved. Most people who have osteoarthritis eventually die from heart-related ailments.

So you should read these facts about eating certain types of fish:

Tuna is one of the fatty fishes which contain EPA and DHA, two very valuable fatty acids. I also recommend salmon, mackerel, trout, shad and sardines.

One $3\frac{1}{2}$ -ounce can of sardines can supply 40 per cent of the daily protein needed by an adult. Salmon and mackerel are very rich in calcium, the bone-building nutrient which helps prevent osteoporosis. (For more about this disease, see Chapter XXI.)

It is interesting to note that the Japanese have rampant high blood pressure, but they have fewer heart attacks than most nationalities. Why? Perhaps it's because the Japanese subsist largely on fish – fatty fish that swim in the colder seas.

Shellfish are considered to be low in fat, but the fat that they do contain has a high proportion of beneficial omega-3 fatty acids.

Every year, the average American eats 13 pounds of fish. But, by comparison, their annual consumption of meat totals 100 pounds per person.

If it is important to you to eat foods which are very low in cholesterol, then enjoy scallops, mussels, oysters and clams. They say fish is 'brain food'. So, get smart. Eat fish!

The Future: New Methods To Test My Dietary Program

I have such confidence in nutrition -- and in cod liver oil – that I am willing to cooperate with any group of scientists or doctors who wish to review my work.

Let's conduct tests, with human patients. I am proposing that a formal clinical evaluation be made.

New medical equipment has been invented in recent years. There is now modern technology that is even more accurate than the gas chromatography which charted the progress of the arthritic patients in London.

I urge scientists to use every device available, and every new technique, to prove whether I am right or wrong.

This is an open invitation to the medical world. Or call it a challenge, if you wish. Let's end the skepticism and dubious remarks.

Personally, I have already started to arrange a clinical

evaluation – which could prove my theories conclusively. I am suggesting that actual biopsies be performed on patients who have serious cases of arthritis.

I am currently conferring with rheumatologists and surgeons in California, trying to assemble a group of their arthritic patients who would take part in this controlled study.

Research into cod liver oil and arthritis has continued and continues to this day. Although responses to dietary changes vary from one arthritis sufferer to another, the effectiveness of fish oils is now well accepted among rheumatologists and sufferers are routinely advised to increase their omega-3 intake.

In the 1950s, Dale Alexander's 'cod liver oil campaign' attracted considerable criticism from the medical fraternity. But the publicity arising from the controversy provoked sufficient interest for two doctors to conduct a scientifically acceptable study using the Alexander method. To the surprise of everyone, with the exception of Dale Alexander himself, nearly every patient studied showed a distinct improvement. The study, published in 1959 in the *Journal of the National Medical Association*, reported as follows: 98 cases of osteo, rheumatoid and mixed arthritis were treated. 92 cases responded within a period of 2 to 20 weeks. The patients themselves noted a marked reduction in pain with a general improvement recorded by the majority.

In 1985 benefits of fish oil supplementation were described in a study by Kremer *et al.* They reported that patients with rheumatoid arthritis had significantly less pain and less morning stiffness after 12 weeks. In 1987 a follow-up trial involving larger doses of fish oil showed that after 14 weeks patients consuming the fish oil exhibited significant improvement, with fewer tender and swollen joints. Similar results were obtained in a 1988 study by Cleland *et al* after 12 weeks. Later studies (der Tempel *et al* 1990 and Tulleken *et al* 1990) confirmed that fish oil supplementation produced clinical improvements in arthritis patients. In 1992 another study demonstrated that patients needed less anti-inflammatory medication.

If fish oils have been proven to help arthritis sufferers, why are doctors so reluctant to recommend this natural treatment over drugs that produce unpleasant side-effects? In my view, the answer lies in the time it takes to effect an improvement. Doctor and patient alike are reluctant to cut back on painkilling drugs for the time it takes for the fish oil to take effect. If you have been prescribed NSAIDs for your arthritis but are unhappy with the way they make you feel, why not ask your doctor if you could try taking cod liver oil and gradually cut down your dependence on the drugs?

Arthroplastic surgeons are certainly qualified to take biopsies while they are operating on patients to replace hip joints or knee joints.

Yes, I urge that biopsies be done. In fact, in addition, let's examine patients with an arthroscope.

Joint linings can now be inspected, inside the human body, by inserting an arthroscopic device. It is a rigid fiberoptic rod-lens telescope. An incision is made (near the afflicted knee joint, for example) and the arthroscope goes in to look around.

This technique is a new one, totally reliable as a diagnostic procedure. The arthroscope apparatus was only an idea a few years ago. Now, it has been manufactured as a modern scientific tool.

There are two Japanese doctors who deserve full credit for inventing the arthroscope. Dr. M. Watanabe and Dr. S. Takeda made medical history by giving the world such a valuable piece of equipment. It can be widely used, to benefit arthritics everywhere.

To gain added knowledge, a tiny camera can be attached to the arthroscope. Pictures of the intra-articular structure can be flashed on a TV screen. Now we can have photographic documentation of how joints look. Let's compare the arthritic joints of patients who follow my diet, with those who don't.

Further, I propose that a series of tests be made by aspirating fluid from joint cavities. With a needle, fluid is drawn from the afflicted joint. My followers, who have been eating oil-bearing foods, will have synovial fluid that is clearer, healthier.

As final proof, the most conclusive test can be the taking of biopsies. A forceps can be attached to the arthroscope, which will enable the surgeon to snip tissue from the synovial membrane or from the cartilage. Give the tissue specimen to a pathologist, so he can study it under a microscope.

I am confident that biopsies will prove, beyond any doubt, that joint linings benefit from cod liver oil.

Those patients who have followed my diet will have better linings. There will be less infiltration of white blood cells, less inflammation and less susceptibility to infection.

Then, perhaps, the medical world will accept the logical truth. It is possible, through correct diet, to build up the viscosity of joint linings. Athritic joints can be self-lubricated to alleviate pain.

Let there be no uncertainty I am proposing that a complete clinical evaluation be made: a controlled study, using two groups of patients, comparing one against the other.

Take biopsies three separate times. Once at the start of the experiment. Then, 20 weeks later, the same patients would be tested again. And, to chart the lasting results, a third set of biopsies would monitor the patients a full year later.

As this chapter has shown, many scientists have made sincere efforts to authenticate my theories. I am most grateful to them, and I pledge to you that testing will continue.

Any 'new' approach to help conquer any disease is questioned, at first. And that's how it should be. I offer full cooperation to medical authorities. Test my dietary program on actual patients. I have abiding faith in the results, past, present, and future.

Chapter XVIII

New Medical Discoveries –
Some Encouraging News

While I was toiling in the field of nutrition, other men and women were achieving significant progress in scientific laboratories. Their accomplishments deserve worldwide attention.

This chapter will express my admiration for those unsung heroes . . . they are conducting experiments night and day, yet their efforts are seldom known to the public.

You, as an arthritic, ought to be told about their research work. Your life and well-being will be vitally affected by these medical pioneers.

For example, do you realize the full impact of the recent discoveries made by immunologists?

Very few people understand 'the immune system' which exists in the human body. It is hard to read any newspaper article which talks about 'the biology of suppressor T-cells' or 'the immunological value of antibodies'.

Perhaps I can clarify some of this technical language, because your future health may be changed dramatically by T-cell and B-cell research. The tests are being done, now . . . and the news is heartening for all arthritics.

Just remember one fact: inside your body, you have approximately one trillion white blood cells. About 100,000,000,000,000,000 are antibody molecules.

The letter 'T' stands for thymus – the thymus gland which manufactures T-cells.

The human body also has other lymphocytes which are

called B-cells – 'B' for bone marrow, where these cells are made.

When a virus or harmful bacteria invades your body, both the T-cells and B-cells react. They produce antibodies to 'kill' the invader.

For instance, let's use the example of crippling rheumatoid arthritis. When a hip joint or knee joint is becoming inflamed (and then infected) your T-cells and B-cells try to counteract that distress. The cells 'make' specific antibodies for that portion of your body. If you have been eating properly, your system can manufacture enough antibodies to save your health.

This is the viewpoint I am trying to impart to scientists everywhere. I respect them, for the research they are doing on T-cells and B-cells. But I wish they would place more emphasis on the patient's diet.

Intestinal Bypass Operations: Too Severe!

Some people with arthritis are also overweight. They have a condition which is now called 'morbid obesity', and surgery is one purported way to end this affliction.

Can you imagine having an intestinal bypass, just to lose those extra pounds? In recent years, we have all heard about the heart 'bypass'. This has now become a favorite option for cardiovascular patients. Even double and triple bypass operations are quite common these days.

But don't listen to anyone who proposes that you have an intestinal bypass. The surgeon would perform this technique on your ileum, the last part of your small intestine. All this, just to combat obesity?

A better way to control your weight is through proper diet. It would be far easier to follow the menus in this book, much more pleasant.

Let me add that a study was done, among actual patients, in

1982. I have read the report, entitled 'Rheumatoid Arthritis Following The Reactive Arthritis Of Bypass Disease.'

In this report, the doctors had to admit one devastating fact. Nine of the patients came down with rheumatoid arthritis after the operation!

This operation has been refined since Dale Alexander warned about such drastic surgery. Although I am of his mind on the undesirability of surgical intervention, in some cases the morbidly overweight are quite unable to lose excess fat by diet. There are heartbreaking examples of people who are so overweight they cannot lead anything approaching a normal life and the prognosis is an early death. In these cases, but only in these, surgery may be the only answer.

Malnutrition is not always synonymous with starvation. These people are malnourished because they have an unhealthy relationship with food. Obesity is a disease of the Western world and is increasing. We must educate our children on food values, on buying and cooking natural produce to share and enjoy with friends and family.

A Safe And Sane Remedy: The Old Reliable!

Why are we discussing new and extreme measures, like bypass surgery, when the best answer to arthritis is readily available in your own home?

Cod liver oil is the natural product which can trigger your recovery. You already know it is not a new discovery . . . the medicinal value of this oil has been established for centuries.

Throughout this book, I have sung the praises of cod liver oil as a source of vitamins. Now, in the next chapter, I want to emphasize one more reason why this extract from codfish can improve your health.

My next topic, is osteoporosis. For people who have weakened bones, cod liver oil can help you maintain the correct balance of calcium and phosphorus in your body.

Chapter XIX

When Bones Begin To Break: That's Osteoporosis!

Every time you visit a convalescent home, you can't help but notice the many people in wheelchairs. And your heart goes out to all those elderly inmates who are walking with crutches.

Brittle bones have become broken bones. It is estimated that once you have passed the age of 60, then 90 per cent of all fractures are due to osteoporosis.

Many victims of hip fractures soon develop other complications – shock, hemorrhaging, etc. – which prove fatal. In fact, osteoporosis has now become the twelfth leading cause of death in the United States.

Some scientists at the Mayo Clinic now believe that two types of osteoporosis exist. They categorize the illness by age group.

Among women, from 50 to 65 years of age, it is known as post-menopausal osteoporosis.

Men and women over the age of 75 suffer from senile osteoporosis.

In all cases, the affliction affects a person's skeletal structure. It is a deficiency of bone mass. Loss of calcium, in older people, leads to thinning of the bones and increased fragility.

Young people, when they are barely 20 years old, make dietary mistakes. This disease really starts to develop at that early age. Prevention is possible, if you read these next few pages.

While writing this book, I had an opportunity to watch a certain television program on the subject of osteoporosis.

The telecast featured two doctors, both of whom are highly educated in regard to this illness. I have known Dr. Arnold Pike for more than 20 years. He is the TV host and commentator who is seen every week on stations coast to coast. Dr. Pike holds a half-hour discussion on topics of health with guests from every field of medicine. It is called *Campus Profile.*

Dr. Pike himself is Director of the Academy of Nutritional Sciences. His TV program is shown in Los Angeles (ABC-TV, Channel 7). (I have appeared on his telecast several times to report my research findings on arthritis.)

Recently, one entire program conducted by Dr. Pike was devoted to a special interview with an expert on osteoporosis. This distinguished guest was Dr. Frank W. Varese. This renowned Italian physician received his M.D. at the University of Bologna.

Dr. Varese came to America in 1968, and he has been practicing internal medicine in this country ever since. He is now a member of the American Academy of Medical Preventics.

(Incidentally, here and now, I would like to praise the work of that Academy. They are a group of 500 physicians doing excellent work. They study chronic degenerative diseases of the circulatory system. Their emphasis is on both prevention and treatment. Dr. Varese is particularly interested in osteoporosis.)

When Dr. Varese and Dr. Pike met on the air, the telecast about osteoporosis was a very scholarly interview. They covered all aspects of this ailment, in concise language.

Here are some highlights – actual quotes, which Dr. Pike provided to me, as transcribed from the soundtrack of the television dialogue:

Dr. Varese: Osteoporosis is a very insidious and frequently crippling disease. It is the most common metabolic disease of the bones.

In lay language, we call it 'thinning of bones'.

Many experts in the medical field like to speak of osteoporosis as 'the silent disease'. Silent, because in many instances a patient has no symptoms whatsoever. The first symptom may be a fracture, a hip fracture.

Dr Pike: What's happening to the bones, in osteoporosis?

Dr. Varese: It's a wasting problem. Bones lose substance, lose mass. A patient can lose as much as 40 per cent to 50 per cent of the total bone mass.

Why? The usual and normal metabolism of bones is disturbed, due to multi-factorial problems – having to do with nutrition, with hormones, life style. Therefore, these bones become weaker, thinner, and frequently collapse. We have a fracture of the vertebrae, fracture of the wrist bone, or fracture of the hip bone.

Dr. Pike: We see a loss of calcium to bones?

Dr. Varese: Yes, there is a loss of calcium. Therefore, bones are not able to give support to the body, and they fracture easily.

Dr. Pike: Why does this occur so commonly as we grow older?

Dr. Varese: As we get older everything occurs more commonly. Osteoporosis actually begins at age 20, and we see the evidence of the disease in older people.

For instance, in women alone (of age 45 and older) every year 200,000 suffer fractures – and, of these, 45,000 die as a consequence.

It is a total disease, for instance, when you discuss cost. Medical expenses, for the fracture of a hip, for the first seven days, can be as high as $14,000! That doesn't take into consideration the follow-up of convalescent homes, physical therapy, etc.

Dr. Pike: So, the consequence of poor diet – as we are ageing – can be of considerable expense to you in the matter of your bones.

Considerable expense? What an understatement! Medical costs are so incredibly high these days, it's a major worry for every arthritic. That TV program, on osteoporosis, did not include any cost estimates for other forms of arthritis.

Suppose, for example, you have rheumatoid pains – to the point where you can suffer no longer. You decide to have surgery. Arthroplasty, to replace a knee joint, costs a small fortune! To escape an avalanche of medical bills caused by osteoporosis you need to know two main facts:

1.   Calcium is the most important factor. Do everything possible to maintain high levels of calcium in your body. Eat calcium-bearing foods.
2.   Estrogen (oestrogen) is a hormone which can help reduce the 'thinning' of bones. Your body can manufacture its own supply of this hormone. Here's how:

Estrogen: Yours For Free, Through Proper Diet

For many years, doctors have instructed their patients to purchase estrogen tablets. This has been the prescribed remedy for patients who were fighting off osteoporosis.

Women often experience a deficiency of estrogen, especially after menopause. Scientific studies have shown that this hormone can sometimes prevent spinal fractures and strengthen bones.

Synthetic estrogen has long been used to reduce 'hot flushes' during menopause. Now, in regard to osteoporosis, this same hormone can be beneficial. But why buy it? Why gulp down expensive tablets? It is a proven fact that your body can easily make its own natural estrogen.

Internally, your system can create hormones – including

estrogen – in abundant supply. You can self-generate more estrogen with the help of Vitamin D.

Your adrenal glands are instrumental in making hormones. It is possible to stimulate your adrenals. They can be 'triggered' into greater action.

Hormone replacement therapy (HRT) is now widely accepted for the relief of menopausal symptoms and to protect against the loss of bone mass that occurs when estrogen production slows down. Many women of menopausal age demand it as a result of its publicized health benefits and because it also has the reputation of prolonging a youthful appearance. However, it is linked with an increased incidence of cancer of the breast and uterus, heart disease and stroke. As HRT is a fairly new treatment there are also concerns about its long-term use. HRT can sigificantly upset the internal balance of natural hormones. Also, it does not suit all women. Calcium supplements are promoted for the maintenance of bone strength, but calcium alone is not enough. Look for calcium malate supplements and include magnesium and Vitamin D (as found in cod liver oil!). Omega-3 and omega-6 fatty acids are essential for the manufacture of prostaglandins, which figure in all hormonal activity and it is important to ensure your intake of these too.

Rickets – This Ailment Is Not Limited To Children!

Since we are discussing the whole spectrum of illnesses which 'soften' bones and disfigure human bodies, I should certainly comment on rickets.

It has touched your heart and mine. You feel compassion whenever you see a bow-legged child. We are sorry for the youngster who must go through life with legs that are bent out of shape.

Through the years, this affliction has been so common, it is listed in *Webster's Dictionary:*

Rickets – a disease of the skeletal system. Resulting from absence of the normal effect of Vitamin D in depositing calcium salts in the bone.

Medical science established this fact – proved the importance of Vitamin D as an antidote for rickets – during experiments performed more than 60 years ago. Working among children, Dr. Ruth Guy was a pioneer in this field in the 1920's. She was a physician, using facilities at Yale University. (See page 21.)

Simultaneously, another group of scientists and pediatricians were making headway against rickets by conducting tests at Johns Hopkins University. Their efforts, in the city of Baltimore, were designed to prove the relative effectiveness of cod liver oil as contrasted with butter fat for protecting the body against insufficient calcium.

The experts at Johns Hopkins reported their key results in *The American Journal of Hygiene.* The title of their medical paper was 'Studies on Experimental Rickets'. Published in June of 1921, it was reprinted for a second time in *Nutrition Reviews,* May 1984. Point: these ideas – theirs, and mine – are not a new, untested theory.

The medical team, in Baltimore, did a series of animal experiments. They fed groups of rats on two separate diets. A mixture of butter fat was added to the food eaten by one set of rats. Another set was given food containing cod liver oil.

Those rats which were raised on a diet that contained butter fat failed to grow normally. They developed a severe rickets-like condition. Some of them became permanently stunted.

Meanwhile, other rats were given the same food – with cod liver oil added. They stayed healthy, fertile, reproducing offspring.

The scientists published their conclusions:

Cod liver oil contains a regulating substance which exerts a profound influence on the behavior of the bone corpuscles and perhaps on other tissues of the body as well.

Without Vitamin D, calcium will not be laid down as strong, healthy bone. It is easier to obtain calcium than Vitamin D from a varied diet, so expert advice for people whose skin is seldom exposed to sunlight, is to take Vitamin D in supplement form. Over recent decades a wealth of evidence has documented Vitamin D deficiency in elderly populations. A daily intake of 800 IU (20mcg) can be obtained from 20ml (one tablespoon plus one teaspoon, or two dessertspoons) of cold liver oil.

As recently as 1998 the British Medical Journal published 'Vitamin D deficiency: time for action' calling for routine Vitamin D supplementation for the elderly and others at risk. There is a wealth of evidence documenting Vitamin D deficiency in Europe, the US and elsewhere.

Osteomalacia – Now Being Called 'Senile Rickets'

Softening of the bones is the primary symptom. This illness strikes older people, but, in some ways, it compares to having rickets in childhood.

If your doctor suspects that you have osteomalacia, he will usually complete his diagnosis by taking a bone biopsy. He may find that the organic matrix of bone has not undergone calcification.

Serum calcium may be reduced. Your serum phosphate (your supply of phosphorus) may be decreased. And your hydroxycholecalciferol levels are reduced to below normal levels.

To recover your health, how can you build up your body's supply of cholecalciferol? Vitamin D_3 is found in cod liver oil. The '3' following the 'D' is the scientific symbol for cholecalciferol.

So, again, to repair softening bones, I am perfectly correct in recommending that you add cod liver oil to your diet.

Dowager's Hump – Shoulders Stooped, Neck Bent Down

You have probably seen some poor woman who seems to be leaning forward, crippled into a painful posture, forced to stare at the ground.

The cause, again, is lack of calcium, weakened bones. The patient has had continued collapse and crush fractures of dorsal and lumbar vertebrae. The areas between the vertebrae in the spine have shrunken. As a result, the person has actually lost height. The victim, physically, is three inches shorter than ever before. The damage can be that great.

Take measures now so that 'dowager's hump' never wrecks your life. Select your foods and menus more carefully.

For all types of osteoporosis, I recommend a specific group of foods which are rich in calcium. Remember, you must eat properly to obtain at least 800 milligrams of calcium each day.

The best sources of calcium are: Green leafy vegetables, such as broccoli, kale, and turnip greens. Egg yolk and soybeans are helpful. Drink milk, and eat fish. When possible, you should also eat the roots or tubers of the green vegetables.

Earlier in this chapter, we discussed the need for natural estrogen. To 'trigger' your adrenal glands – to make more and better estrogen within your body – you must increase your intake of Vitamin D.

The three most productive food sources of this oil-soluble vitamin are: whole milk (when the fat is taken out of the milk, the fat-soluble Vitamins A and D go with it), eggs, and cod liver oil.

Don't worry, you can avoid the 'taste' factor. Modern technology has created emulsified cod liver oil. It is pleasant to take, literally tasteless.

For victims of osteoporosis only, I now suggest that you consume your cod liver oil from a spoon. Do not mix it with milk or orange juice. You should take one tablespoon of emulsified cod liver oil each day, 30 minutes before breakfast.

If you already have osteoporosis, that means you have drained the calcium reserves from your bones. It can become a life-threatening problem that goes far beyond the minor relief you can gain by taking synthetic estrogen. I repeat, make your own natural estrogen – as described above.

By observing my dietary plan, which I have set forth throughout this book, you can achieve good health. Otherwise, what happens? Turn this page.

Chapter XX

Surgery For Arthritis: The Price You Pay

If pain, inflammation and stiffness continue unabated, you can't just ignore your arthritis. Don't sit around waiting for some miraculous remission. Either take some remedial steps, now – or you may have to telephone a surgeon and check into a hospital.

Surgery is a harrowing experience, physically and financially. Even so, many arthritics now subject themselves to major operations. For example, a stainless steel plate can be implanted into the femur bone of the knee. The lower bone (the tibia) is given a new plastic component made of polyethylene.

A successful operation of this type serves the arthritic patient in four ways. Surgery can:

1. Relieve pain in the joint.
2. Restore function.
3. Arrest destruction of the joint.
4. Correct deformities, and improve the appearance of deformed joints.

Yes, these are important advantages for a victim of arthritis. The success rate – for partial or total replacement of joints – has been high. Therefore, in this chapter, I shall give you the latest facts about this surgical procedure. You can then decide whether arthroplasty should be in your plans for the future.

I have known many individuals who were confined to wheel-chairs. But now they are walking again, thanks to arthroplastic surgery.

Among all these case histories, I shall always remember one lady whom I met in Edinburgh, Scotland. She had eight plastic fingers, two plastic hips, and two plastic knees. She had been 'reconstructed' so often, you might call her 'The Bionic Woman'.

Most important, this middle-aged arthritic was now living a happy, pain-free life. She attended one of my lectures, in Scotland, and I talked with her at length about arthroplasty.

Upon returning to the United States, I resumed my research into these surgical techniques. I am very favorably impressed by the post-operative recovery that arthritics report.

The future for orthopedic surgery is bright, as surgeons will be introducing artificial joints which are made of better materials. One expert who is predicting revolutionary developments in this field is Dr. James R. Klinenberg.

Dr. Klinenberg is a clinical professor of medicine at UCLA School of Medicine and is also chairman of the Department of Medicine at Cedar Sinai Medical Center.

The widespread acceptance of surgery for arthritics has impressed many doctors. Today, in America, there are more than 12,000 orthopedic surgeons, and many of them have become specialists in arthroplasty.

All these activities – the expansion of surgical aid for arthritics – can be traced back to discoveries made by one man. The principal inventor of mechanical joints was Dr. John Charnley. He conducted years of experiments, in England.

Surgeons everywhere credit Dr. Charnley as being the originator of modern total hip arthroplasty. He developed this medical procedure, emphasizing the low friction principle: utilizing metal against plastic to create an artificial joint.

The major part of his work took place during the 1970s. His contribution to medical science was so great, the Queen of England made him a Commander of the British Empire. He became Sir John Charnley, respected by rheumatologists around the world.

To write this chapter – in order to give you correct facts – I set out to find an outstanding surgeon who could answer my questions. In America, a recognized authority on arthroplasty is Dr. Leonard Marmor. In medical circles, his book is a classic. Entitled: *Arthritis Surgery*, it is required reading for many young doctors.

Dr. Marmor has personally performed more than 900 hip replacements and 500 knee replacements. Today, he is attending surgeon at St. John's Hospital in Santa Monica.

I met with Dr. Marmor, and we discussed the latest arthroplasty techniques. We talked about synovial fluid, cartilage, the risks of infection, and a wide range of topics. I sincerely appreciate the way Dr. Marmor shared his wisdom.

How popular has arthroplastic surgery become? Or, rather, how necessary are these operations? To many arthritics, tortured by constant pain, surgery is the only solution they can find.

Today, far too many people must seek this form of help. Arthroplasty now ranks among the top 20 surgical procedures performed in the United States. Because of the frequency of these operations, that's a sad record to hold.

Equally grim – in terms of human suffering – is the fact that more people than ever before are checking into hospitals because they have serious knee damage.

The bad news roster continues and we must add all the operations on arthritic elbows, plus arthroplasty to repair crippled fingers.

Now Hear This: Lecture Given By A Famous Scientist

It was an historic speech, a landmark lecture on the topic of arthroplasty.

The talk was delivered in England by Professor J. H.

Kellgren, director of the Rheumatism Research Centre at Manchester University.

He began by defining osteoarthritis in anatomical terms as 'a softening, fibrillation, and eventual disintegration of articular cartilage, resulting in joint-narrowing.'

Professor Kellgren then stated that 'the essence of a good arthroplasty was that the resulting joint have a low coefficient of friction.'

He commented about the use of intra-articular injections as lubricants in 'creaky' joints. The professor pointed out that:

> Even if desirable, it was impractical, since the injections would have to be repeated with great frequency. In any event, the joint fluid in osteoarthritis was generally of a good quality – that is, of high viscosity and consisting of highly polymerized hyaluronic acid.

As reported in the *British Medical Journal*, Professor Kellgren did not feel that muscle relaxants had any place in treatment, since, although the stiffness might appear to come from the muscles, most of the symptoms arose from the joints and periarticular tissues, which could not be affected by such drugs.

Professor Kellgren is yet another expert whose views are very close to mine. His facts match statements I have made for years.

Now that you know the history of arthroplasty, you may have less fear of being hospitalized. Nobody likes to take that lonely ride on a gurney into the operating room. But sometimes surgery is justified, and arthritics can gain dramatic improvement.

The surgical techniques which began in England (with Sir John Charnley) have been refined and perfected. They are now widely accepted.

Patients now ask for arthroplasty, which is much preferred over arthrodesis. You should note and remember the difference.

Arthrodesis is surgical fusion of a joint. Instead of binding an arthritic joint into a solid state, arthroplasty can restore movement and near normal function.

Your chances to gain relief will soon increase. Results have been good involving hips and knees. Now research is underway whereby arthroplasty can be used for total replacement of ankle joints.

Total shoulder arthroplasty is also in the design stage. Early results in a few patients are considered encouraging.

In this chapter, perhaps I have sounded very enthusiastic about arthroplastic surgery. I do favor the technique – but I am not too happy about sending any arthritic to a hospital.

It saddens me when anyone neglects his or her body to a point where only a surgeon's scalpel can solve the problem. If you correct your eating habits now, you can avoid arthroplasty. It's your choice. You can reconstruct your diet – or be reconstructed.

Chapter XXI

Cholesterol: Some Conclusive Comments

Are you confused by the controversy which has been raging on the topic of cholesterol? I don't blame you for wondering. There has been a flood of newspaper articles as many different doctors make conflicting statements in this 'pro and con' debate.

In these last few pages of my book, perhaps the greatest service I can render to my readers is to write about cholesterol. Here's what I believe are the latest and most definitive facts.

The most reliable medical report on cholesterol – the one you can trust – is The Framingham Study. A total of 5,127 men and women between the ages of 30 and 60 (all residents of Framingham, Massachusetts) have been examined biennially for 34 years. They have had their cholesterol levels monitored since 1949!

For the results, worth reading, I called Doctor William P. Castelli, Medical Director at the National Heart, Lung and Blood Institute in Framingham.

You can improve the ratio between polyunsaturated oils and saturated oils in your system only if you pay close attention as to how and when you drink water. In your battle to correct the levels of cholesterol in your body, please observe the water and beverage-drinking rules which I detailed on pages 96 through 101.

Most adults, on the average, have a cholesterol level of between 200mg per cent to 250mg per cent per 100 cc's of blood serum. I believe that a better ratio would be to keep your level between 175mg per cent to 200mg per cent. Proper diet can accomplish this goal.

Within your body there are two kinds of cholesterol. One type is made up of high-density lipoproteins, and you also have a supply of low-density lipoproteins.

I maintain that you can and should increase your bodily supply of high-density lipoproteins, and ingesting cod liver oil is one good way to do it.

If I were teaching in a college, a cornerstone of my course on Nutrition would concern the ill-effects of water when it is consumed with meals. Everyone must be educated on how to protect the lipids (the oils) which exist in your body.

You must learn to change the function of these lipids. In the past, the emphasis has always been that lipids serve as fuel. In the future, let's learn how to eat and drink so that the lipids can bypass your liver and become lubricants. This is how to manufacture favorable prostaglandins.

As a foremost weapon in this dietary plan, I can again recommend cod liver oil. This type of oil can act as a lesion-repairing substance in coronary arteries.

In some areas, on the topic of cholesterol, I find myself in agreement with the noted nutritionist Carlton Fredericks. He is not in favor of the Pritikin diet, nor am I. That diet has claimed to build resistance to heart attacks by dramatically reducing cholesterol and saturated fat intakes.

Dr. Fredericks made some excellent points not long ago. Writing in *Let's Live* magazine, he said:

> Cholesterol is essential to life. Many vital processes in the body are dependent upon cholesterol, ranging from the sheaths (myelin) which insulate the nerves, to the manufacture of indispensable hormones, including sex hormones.

Cholesterol continues to generate great interest and controversy. It is now widely accepted that cholesterol is essential and indeed the body produces it as a normal and necessary blood component. It is the balance between HDL (good) and LDL (bad) cholesterol that needs to be maintained for heart health.

As I have explained before, the omega-3 essential fatty acids are powerful allies in the fight against heart disease. Oily fish, fish oils and, of course, cod liver oil are the best and most readily available sources and certainly more valuable than omega-3 oils extracted from vegetables, nuts and seeds.

Although omega-3 DHA and EPA do not lower total cholesterol, they do have a positive effect on the balance between LDL (low-density lipoprotein) and HDL (high-density lipoprotein) by increasing HDL in the blood. HDL is heart protective whereas high LDL levels greatly increase the risk of heart attack.

My Final Exhibit: Proof Beyond Question!

The mounting evidence which strengthens my case – more medical research that confirms my emphasis on proper diet – reached a peak in February of 1985.

The good news originated in Albany, New York, and I soon heard about it in a letter which was mailed to me from Newcastle, England.

Living in Newcastle upon Tyne is a prominent medical writer named Joseph T. McKiernan. I met him in 1979 and again in 1983, when he interviewed me for *The Newcastle Evening Chronicle*.

One day recently, he sent me a wonderful message. He enclosed a clipping from London – from *the Sunday Times*. The headline announced that diet offers new hope to arthritis victims, and the article read:

Researchers have discovered that a diet of fish and lean meat, with fish-oil supplements, reduces stiffness and pain in the joints caused by rheumatoid arthritis.

The discovery was made at Albany Medical College, New York State, after a rigorous trial in which neither doctors nor patients knew who was receiving active treatment and who was being given a dummy course.

The results, reported in *The Lancet*, are the first scientific evidence that food plays an important part in the disease.

. . . The diet that helped the American patients is similar to that recommended for the prevention of heart disease.

. . . After three months on the Albany diet, patients had fewer tender joints and suffered less stiffness than others who had been on a standard American diet high in saturated fat. When they were taken off the polyunsaturated diet, the number of tender joints increased.

Let me express my humble thanks to the scientists at the Albany Medical College in New York State. They are recognizing some of the precepts that I have been preaching for 35 years.

This letter, from the medical journalist in Newcastle, I shall always treasure:

Dear Dale:
I nearly fell into the fire when I read the enclosed.

If ever a man was justified in what he said, against all medical opinion, it is you.

Let me have your comments for publication. In my view, you have been completely vindicated.

Yours sincerely,

Joseph T. McKiernan

Increase Your IQ On MS

It's time for all of us to learn more about MS. Multiple sclerosis is a calamity when it strikes, and this disease is spreading in nations throughout the world.

MS, all too often, is appearing in patients who have already contracted arthritis. I experienced a shocking example of this trend when I was in Cardiff, Wales, not long ago. I was being interviewed on a Cardiff radio station. Listeners were telephoning questions to me on the air. That day I was besieged with calls which all began with the same bad news: 'I have arthritis and multiple sclerosis! Why? What causes this double trouble?'

The answers I gave during that radio broadcast were crucially important. To help prevent MS, I should repeat my views now, in this book.

A person suffering from MS is also a victim of dryness. Lack of lubrication within the human body can lead to serious damage throughout your nervous system.

Thanks to medical science it is now possible to diagnose multiple sclerosis during the early stages of the illness. (The method to detect MS is known as the E-UFA tests – an analysis involving unsaturated fatty acids.) MS affects the brain, the spinal cord, and nerve fibers in many areas of your body. If you can hardly walk (and must drag either foot) that could be MS. You may have pain in your hand. That pins-and-needles sensation is one symptom of MS.

You might feel the effects of MS in your hand or foot, but actually these problems are due to damage which has occurred in your central nervous system.

Each nerve fiber is surrounded by a layer of 'insulation' composed mainly of fatty material that is called myelin. Loss of myelin – through faulty diet? – destroys the ability of your nerves to conduct impulses from your brain.

This 'drying-out' process starts to happen in many areas of your body simultaneously, so physicians began to describe the illness as 'multiple' sclerosis. Dryness sets in, then lesions develop. To repair these lesions, your body forms a crust or scar in your central nervous system. The term 'sclerosis' means scarring – and no wonder your nerves can't function properly!

To protect the lubricating myelin which forms a sheath around your nerve fibers, start paying attention to the liquids you drink. Caustic beverages are your enemy. Defend yourself against MS, by correcting your drinking habits.

For example, in regard to this disease, I told those radio listeners in Cardiff that their MS problems were aggravated because they drank too much tea. Those Welsh people imbibe too many cups of black and green tea. They demyelinate themselves with harmful tannic acid.

MS In America – The Citrus Syndrome
Senior citizens living in Florida often complain of painful ailments which could be identified as multiple sclerosis. Anyone who consumes copious quantities of citrus juices may someday suffer the agonies of MS.

Recently, I gave a series of four lectures in Miami Beach. In each audience there were people who had dual diseases – they were afflicted with arthritis and MS. To combat both ailments I urged them to avoid beverages which have a high content of acetic and citric acids.

At one of my lectures, in Florida, someone in the audience asked specifically about apple juice. I replied that apple juice is a lipolytic liquid. It destroys fats and oils which your body needs as a safeguard against MS.

When you drink the juice of an apple, it goes down too quickly, with no time to mix with your saliva. Therefore, your skin and your nerve tissues must neutralize the acid. Your saliva could have done the job properly. The better method is to eat an apple. Chew it thoroughly. Let your saliva be the neutralizer.

Author's note: To help more people escape the misery of multiple sclerosis, I shall continue studying this disease – and I'll report my opinions during future lectures. Much of my knowledge about this illness was gathered in personal meetings I have had with doctors and scientists. Among the experts I have consulted are two of the world's foremost authorities on MS. Next month, I shall travel to Great Britain, where I will meet with them again.

I am grateful for the insight which was given to me by Dr. Michael Crawford, a biochemist at the Nuffield Laboratories of Comparative Medicine in London. I am also indebted to Dr. E. J. Field, famed for his work in the Multiple Sclerosis Research Unit at the Royal Victoria Infirmary, Newcastle upon Tyne. Thank you, gentlemen!

And Finally . . .

I end on a lighter note. I once read a poem by Stephen Vincent Benét. Yes, he wrote some poetry about arthritis. These lines:

> You do not shoot the doctor,
> even when he looks perplexed,
> And you wonder rather dolefully,
> just what is coming next.
> From a weekly dose of gold salts,
> to a jacket made of tin –

Just swallow down your aspirin,
and take it on the chin.

I envy a poet who can write humorously about arthritis. To me, this illness is far too serious. Seldom can I smile.

America, as a nation, is suffering the results. Arthritis is a costly blow to our economy. For you, however, arthritis is a personal and painful problem. If your joints ache, all you want to know is some method of relief.

I hope this book has offered you encouragement, knowledge, and some valid ideas you can act upon.

As for me, my work has only begun. There is more research to be performed; millions of people who must be convinced that nutrition is best. I sincerely believe that these pages hold the most practical answer to arthritis.

Perhaps, someday, colleges and universities around the world will teach dietary techniques to prevent disease. I'll make a prophecy: the day is coming when educational institutions will establish a Chair of Nutrition as part of their academic program.

Another prediction: by the turn of the century, my theories about 'osmosis' and oil-bearing foods may become known as the Law of Assimilation. It may be accepted as medical fact.

Meanwhile, you now have all the facts necessary. You can make a beginning, or ignore them. But you know what? I trust your common sense.

The Last Word

To everything Dale Alexander has written about cod liver oil, I would like to add that every year science discovers more reasons why this humble liquid should be included in everyone's health regime.

Most recently, attention has been focused on the brain.

The omega-3 fatty acid DHA (one of the two fatty acids in cod liver oil) is essential to brain and retina development in the foetus and is recommended to pregnant women in the last three months (third trimester) of pregnancy. It can also make a difference to the new-born baby and many infant formulas are now including fatty acids (found naturally in breastmilk). While on the subject of babies, women on high fish diets or fish oil supplementation produced heavier babies – an indicator of heart health in adulthood.

Other studies link fish oil with asthma, although the benefits are not conclusively proven. Fish oil supplementation is also used following transplants of organs such as kidneys to counteract the side-effects of immunosuppressant drugs.

Cod liver oil itself has also undergone changes since Dale Alexander put down his pen. It has had to ride claims that, as a result of contamination of our oceans, it contains toxins that are detrimental to health. It is a tragedy that the environment is increasingly polluted and therefore much of our fresh food sources are contaminated to some degree. Fish are one such. Fortunately, cod liver oil is subjected to refining processes that remove harmful pollutants. The technological advances that have made it possible to detect even the most minute traces of pollution have been accompanied by refining technology so sophisticated that cod liver oil is safe as well as beneficial to health.

The latest development is also a very positive one. Science has now made it possible to raise levels of the omega-3s in cod liver oil by enriching it with added fish oil concentrate. There is now a wider choice so you can choose the right one for you:

Maintenance: Original cod liver oil supplies vitamins A, D, E and omega-3 fatty acids to maintain general good health and good looks.

Protection: high strength cod liver oil supplies more of the omega-3s for heart health protection.

Therapeutic: extra high strength cod liver oil provides the higher levels of omega-3s required to relieve inflammation, joint pain and stiffness.

Both Vitamin D and the omega-3 DHA and EPA fatty acids are not easy to obtain in a normal diet and I would reiterate that deficiency is certainly not uncommon, particularly among the 50-plus. If you only take one health supplement, make it cod liver oil as this natural oil is a rich source of al lthree nutrients.

Yours in health,
Mark Occhipinti.

If you have found this book helpful, you may be interested in another book on arthritis from Vermilion:

DIET AND ARTHRITIS by Dr Gail Darlington and Linda Gamlin

Co-written by a leading rheumatologist, Dr Gail Darlington, this book looks at the different kinds of arthritis and what causes them. It explains why some diets work for certain arthritic diseases – and why some diets are a waste of time.

009 181659 9 £6.99

Available from all good bookshops or call our mail order hotline number on:
01206 255 800 Postage and packing is free.

More Books from Vermilion

Prices correct at time of going to press

07493 0938 5	**The Courage to Heal**	Ellen Bass and Laura Davis	£10.99
07493 0856 7	**The Body Has Its Reason: Anti-exercise and Self-Awareness**		
		Therese Bertherat and Carol Bernstein	£4.99
07493 0579 7	**How to Develop Self-Confidence and Influence People by Public Speaking**	Dale Carnegie	£7.99
07493 0593 2	**How to Enjoy Your Life and Your Job**	Dale Carnegie	£7.99
07493 0723 4	**How to Stop Worrying and Start Living**	Dale Carnegie	£7.99
07493 0784 6	**How to Win Friends and Influence People**	Dale Carnegie	£7.99
07493 0577 0	**The Quick and Easy Way to Effective Speaking**	Dale Carnegie	£7.99
07493 0246 1	**Overcoming Overeating**	Jane Hirschmann & Carol Munter	£8.99
07493 0933 4	**The Amazing Results of Positive Thinking**	Norman Vincent Peale	£7.99
07493 1341 2	**Courage and Confidence**	Norman Vincent Peale	£7.99
07493 0719 6	**Inspiring Messages for Daily Living**	Norman Vincent Peale	£6.99
07493 0858 3	**The Positive Way to Change Your Life**	Norman Vincent Peale	£7.99
07493 0821 4	**The Power of Positive Living**	Norman Vincent Peale	£7.99
07493 0715 3	**The Power of Positive Thinking**	Norman Vincent Peale	£7.99
07493 0567 3	**The Power of Positive Thinking for Young People**		
		Norman Vincent Peale	£7.99
07493 0254 2	**Families and How to Survive Them**	Robin Skinner and John Cleese	£6.99
07493 2320 5	**Life and How to Survive It**	Robin Skinner and John Cleese	£7.99
009 181679 3	**Living with ME: A Self Help Guide**	Dr Charles Shepherd	£9.99
07493 1656 X	**Victims No Longer**	Mike Lew	£9.99
07493 2665 4	**The Handbook of Alternative and Complementary Medicine**		
		Stephen Fulder	£12.99
07493 2289 6	**Your Child's Symptoms Explained**	Dr David Haslam	£7.99
07493 0936 9	**The Courage to Grieve**	Judith Tatelbaum	£6.99